NURSING PHOTOBOOK™

Controlling Infection

NURSING81 BOOKS
INTERMED COMMUNICATIONS, INC.
HORSHAM, PENNSYLVANIA

1888
WC100
C 60
1981

NURSING81 BOOKS

NURSING PHOTOBOOK™ SERIES
Providing Respiratory Care
Managing I.V. Therapy
Dealing with Emergencies
Giving Medications
Assessing Your Patients
Using Monitors
Providing Early Mobility
Giving Cardiac Care
Performing GI Procedures
Implementing Urologic Procedures
Controlling Infection
Ensuring Intensive Care
Coping with Neurologic Disorders
Caring for Surgical Patients
Working with Orthopedic Patients
Nursing Pediatric Patients
Helping Geriatric Patients
Attending Ob/Gyn Patients
Aiding Ambulatory Patients
Carrying Out Special Procedures

NURSING SKILLBOOK® SERIES
Reading EKGs Correctly
Dealing with Death and Dying
Managing Diabetics Properly
Assessing Vital Functions Accurately
Helping Cancer Patients Effectively
Giving Cardiovascular Drugs Safely
Giving Emergency Care Competently
Monitoring Fluid and Electrolytes Precisely
Documenting Patient Care Responsibly
Combatting Cardiovascular Diseases Skillfully
Coping with Neurologic Problems Proficiently
Using Crisis Intervention Wisely
Nursing Critically Ill Patients Confidently

NURSE'S REFERENCE LIBRARY™
Diseases

Nursing81 DRUG HANDBOOK™

NURSING PHOTOBOOK™ Series
PUBLISHER
Eugene W. Jackson

EDITORIAL DIRECTOR
Jean Robinson

CLINICAL DIRECTOR
Barbara McVan, RN

ART DIRECTOR
Lisa A. Gilde

**Intermed Communications
Book Division**
DIRECTOR
Daniel L. Cheney

DIRECTOR, RESEARCH
Elizabeth O'Brien

DIRECTOR, PRODUCTION AND PURCHASING
Bacil Guiley

Staff for this volume
BOOK EDITOR
Patricia R. Urosevich

CLINICAL EDITOR
Paulette J. Strauch, RN

ASSOCIATE CLINICAL EDITOR
Mary Horstman Obenrader, RN

ASSOCIATE EDITOR
Sally Nimaroff Sapega

PHOTOGRAPHER
Paul A. Cohen

ASSOCIATE DESIGNERS
Linda Jovinelly Franklin
Carol Stickles

ASSISTANT PHOTOGRAPHER
Thomas Staudenmayer

EDITORIAL/GRAPHIC COORDINATOR
Doreen K. Stowers

CLINICAL/GRAPHIC COORDINATOR
Evelyn M. James

COPY EDITORS
Kathlyn J. Foster
Eric R. Rinehimer

EDITORIAL STAFF ASSISTANT
Cynthia A. O'Connell

PHOTOGRAPHY ASSISTANT
Frank Margeson

ART PRODUCTION MANAGER
Robert Perry

ARTISTS
Lorraine Carbo   Joan Walsh
Diane Fox   Robert Walsh
Sandra Simms   Ron Yablon
Louise Stamper

RESEARCHER
Vonda Heller

TYPOGRAPHY MANAGER
David C. Kosten

TYPOGRAPHY ASSISTANTS
Janice Auch
Nancy Boesch
Ethel Halle
Diane Paluba

PRODUCTION MANAGERS
Robert L. Dean, Jr.
Deborah C. Meiris

PRODUCTION ASSISTANT
Donald G. Knauss

ILLUSTRATORS
Bob Boerner   Marsha Jessup
John Dougherty   Bob Jones
Jean Gardner   Pat Macht
Robert Jackson   Bud Yingling

SERIES GRAPHIC DESIGNER
John C. Isely

COVER PHOTO
Paul A. Cohen

**Clinical consultants
for this volume**

Dorothy Borton, RN, BSN
Infection Control Practitioner
Albert Einstein Medical Center, Northern Division
Philadelphia, Pa.

Nancy P. McNew, RN, BSN
Infection Control Practitioner
Anne Arundel General Hospital
Annapolis, Md.

Copyright © 1981 by Intermed
Communications, Inc.,
132 Welsh Road, Horsham, PA 19044
All rights reserved. Reproduction in
whole or part by any means
whatsoever without written permission
of the publisher is prohibited by law.
Printed in the United States of America.

01881

Library of Congress Cataloging in Publication Data

Main entry under title:

Controlling infection.

  (Nursing Photobook)
  "Nursing81 books."
  Bibliography: p.
  Includes index.
  1. Communicable diseases—Nursing.   2. Asepsis and
antisepsis.   3. Nosocomical infections—Prevention.
  [DNLM: 1. Cross infection—Prevention and control—Nursing
texts.   WX 167 C764]
RT95.C66   614.4'4   81-6601
ISBN 0-916730-35-2   AACR2

Contents

Introduction

Understanding fundamentals

CONTRIBUTORS TO
THIS SECTION INCLUDE:
Deborah R. Bauer, RN, BSN, MCH
Cheryl G. Blane, RN

8 Microbiology
18 Culturing

Preventing infection

CONTRIBUTORS TO
THIS SECTION INCLUDE:
Deborah R. Bauer, RN, BSN, MCH
Loretta Tretina, RN

50 Immunization
59 Environmental considerations
76 Cleaning, disinfecting, and sterilizing

Limiting infection

CONTRIBUTORS TO
THIS SECTION INCLUDE:
Doris M. Furlong, RN
Barbara McVan, RN
Paulette J. Strauch, RN
Loretta Tretina, RN

90 Isolation procedures
106 Antibiotic therapy

Coping with invasive therapy

CONTRIBUTORS TO
THIS SECTION INCLUDE:
Beverly J. Brown, RN, BSN
Joyce Turner, RN, BSN, MSN

112 Percutaneous pathways
138 Surgical wounds
148 External body openings

155 Acknowledgements
156 Selected references
158 Index

Contributors

Deborah R. Bauer is health services supervisor for the Kimberly-Clark Corporation. She received her BSN from the University of Oklahoma, and her MCH from Emory University, Atlanta. She is a member of the Association for Practitioners in Infection Control.

Cheryl G. Blane recently became director of the Infection Control Department of Georgetown University Hospital, Washington D.C., after working as infection control coordinator at Doctors' Hospital of Prince Georges County, Lanham, Maryland. She received her nursing diploma from St. Luke's Hospital School of Nursing, Kansas City, Missouri. She is a member of the local and national branches of the Association for Practitioners in Infection Control, and has attended a training course on "Surveillance, Prevention, and Control of Nosocomial Infections" conducted by the Centers for Disease Control, Atlanta.

Dorothy Borton, adviser to this PHOTOBOOK, is a former infection control practitioner at Albert Einstein Medical Center, Northern Division, Philadelphia. She received her BSN degree from Roberts Wesleyan College, Rochester, New York. She is a member of the Delaware Valley/Philadelphia Chapter of the Association for Practitioners in Infection Control.

Beverly J. Brown, an infection control nurse at the Veterans Administration Medical Center, Dallas, Texas, received her BSN degree from Texas Christian University. She is a member of the Association for Practitioners in Infection Control.

Doris M. Furlong is assistant head nurse, Neonatal Intensive Care Unit, Albert Einstein Medical Center, Northern Division, Philadelphia. She received her nursing diploma from Lankenau Hospital School of Nursing, Philadelphia.

Nancy P. McNew, adviser to this PHOTOBOOK, is an infection control nurse at Anne Arundel General Hospital, Annapolis, Maryland. She received her BSN from Ohio State University, and belongs to the Association for Practitioners in Infection Control.

Loretta Tretina is a nurse epidemiologist at St. Agnes Medical Center in Philadelphia. She earned her nursing diploma from Episcopal Hospital in Philadelphia, and is now pursuing a BS degree in Health Education at Temple University (Philadelphia). She attended the training course "Surveillance, Prevention, and Control of Nosocomial Infections" conducted by the Centers for Disease Control, Atlanta. She is a member of the local and national branches of the Association for Practitioners in Infection Control.

Joyce Turner is a nursing instructor at the Veterans Administration Medical Center, Dallas, Texas. She earned her BSN from Texas Christian University, and her MSN in Psychiatric Nursing from Texas Woman's University.

Introduction

ontrolling infection is everyone's responsibility. No matter where you work—hospital, nursing home, or clinic—the employees, patients, and visitors all play a part in preventing and controlling nosocomial infections.

But, as a nurse, you play the most important role in infection control. Think about it. Hardly a moment passes when you're not identifying, preventing, controlling, or teaching others about infection.

We at NURSING PHOTOBOOKS know that practicing day-to-day infection control can be difficult. Understanding the hows and whys of infection control also is difficult. So, we've consulted microbiologists, epidemiologists, and infection-control practitioners in various hospital settings. Then, with their help, we've written this PHOTOBOOK to give you the practical help you need to meet your infection-control responsibilities.

In easy-to-understand terms and with clear photos, CONTROLLING INFECTION provides what no other infection-control book does. For example, in the first section we tell you how and why an infection develops, how it spreads, and how you can keep it from spreading. We've also included exclusive color illustrations of highly magnified microorganisms and white blood cells to make your understanding easier.

As you look through Section 1, you'll find almost everything you need to know about obtaining a specimen for culture; for example, how to obtain a sputum specimen by nasotracheal suction, and how to properly time taking a blood specimen for culture.

In Section 2, you'll learn how to prevent and cope with infection in the hospital. Specifically, we tell you what immunizations are considered routine, when to report a communicable disease, and how to teach your patient about a food-associated infection. In addition, you'll find tips on choosing a disinfectant, selecting a sterilization method, and cleaning a soiled instrument.

Are you uncertain about isolation precautions? This procedure-packed PHOTOBOOK shows you how to put on a sterile gown, double bag linen, and transport an infected patient. We'll also give you details on how to make isolation less traumatic for your patient and his family.

The last section of this book focuses on aseptic technique. It's all here: inserting a peripheral I.V. line, dressing a draining wound, and emptying a Foley catheter bag. You'll also find lots of nursing tips to make your job easier and help reduce hospital-associated infections.

As you know, properly controlling infection imposes great responsibilities. But, regardless of your health-care facility's size and staffing, you can meet these responsibilities with skill and competence. Use this PHOTOBOOK to guide you.

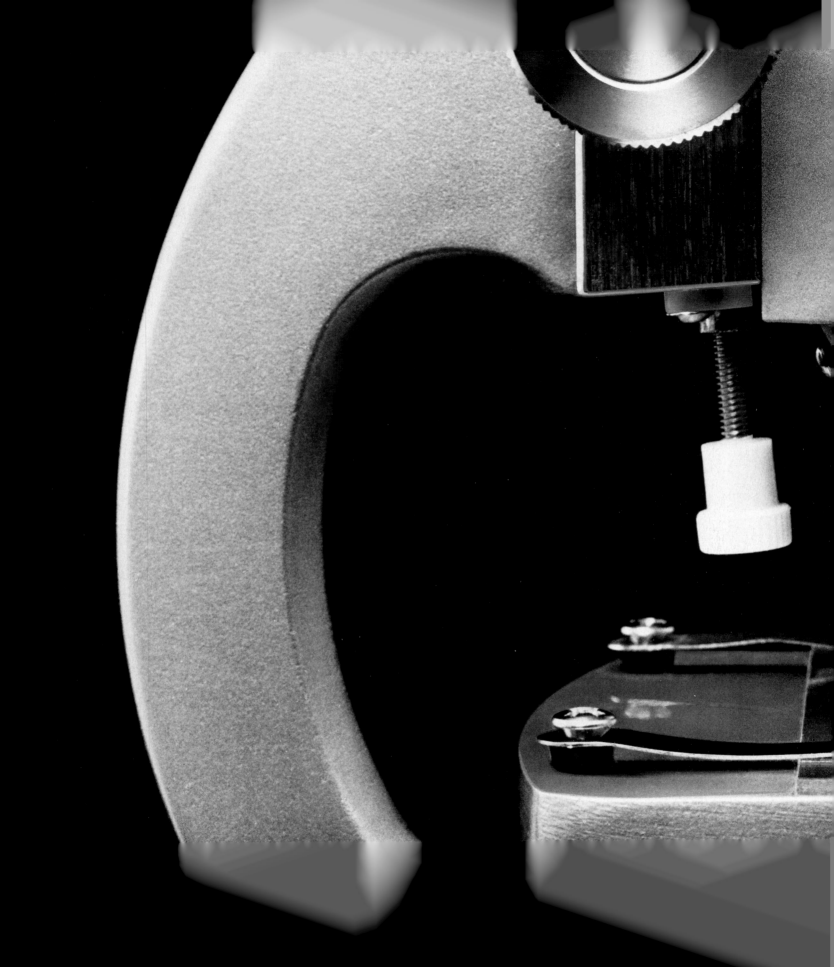

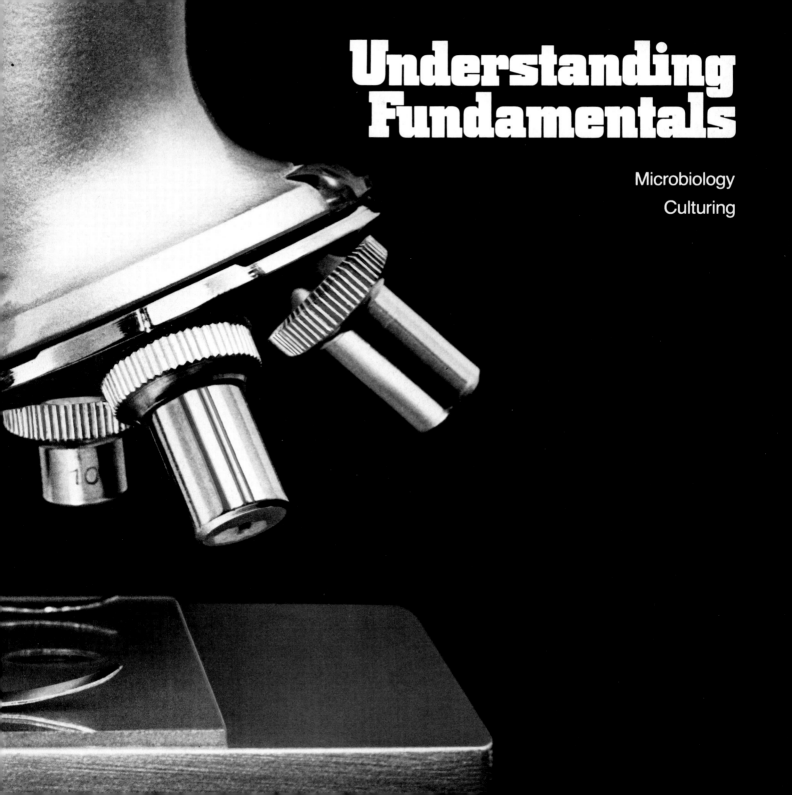

Understanding Fundamentals

Microbiology

Culturing

Microbiology

How much do you know about microbiology? For example, do you know how microorganisms differ? Which microorganisms help the body function? Or, how infection spreads?

If you're like most nurses, you probably haven't studied microbiology for some time. But, reviewing the basics will help you understand infection control. Refresh your memory by reading the next few pages.

Microbiology: Reviewing basic terms

To help you better understand infection control, let's review some definitions of basic terms used in microbiology:

Aerobe: An organism that needs oxygen to survive

Anaerobe: An organism that can't survive when oxygen's present

Carrier: A seemingly healthy person who harbors a disease-causing microorganism

Colonization: Growth of microorganisms in a host without causing a physiologic reaction

Contaminant: A transient harmful microorganism on an animate or inanimate object

Endotoxin: Poisonous substance released from a disintegrated microorganism

Exotoxin: Poisonous substance released from a living microorganism

Host: A living organism that harbors or nourishes a parasite

Infection: Invasion and replication of harmful microorganisms in the body with resulting physiologic response

Nosocomial infection: Invasion and replication of harmful hospital-associated microorganisms in the body with resulting physiologic response

Pathogen: A disease-producing microorganism

Reservoir: A place (animate or inanimate) where harmful microorganisms reside, grow, and multiply

Nurses' guide to microorganisms

Not all microorganisms are alike. But every microorganism can be classified according to size, structure, and mode of transmission.

The chart below describes seven of these major classifications. In addition, we've included common examples of each classification and their effects on man.

Classification and characteristics	Mode of transmission	Examples and effects
Bacteria Unicellular with rigid cell wall; spherical (coccus), rod (bacillus), or spiral (vibrio, spirochete, spirilum) shaped; free living (needs no host to survive)	• Contact • Vector • Common vehicle • Airborne	• *Staphylococcus aureus* (commonly causes boils and wound abscesses) • *Treponema pallidum* (causes syphilis) • *Lactobacillus acidophilus* (aids digestion)
Virus Unicellular with nonrigid cell wall; categorized by animal (spherical shaped), plant (rod shaped or multisided), or bacteriophage (tadpole or rod shaped); needs host to survive.	• Vector • Contact (usually direct or droplet)	• Herpes simplex (causes cold sores) • Tobacco mosaic (causes tobacco-mosaic disease) • Staphylophage (attacks staphylococci)
Chlamydia (formerly Bedsonia) Unicellular with rigid cell wall; spherical shaped; needs host to survive.	• Contact (usually direct or droplet) • Airborne	• *Chlamydia trachomatis* (causes trachoma) • *Chlamydia psittaci* (causes psittacosis)
Mycoplasma Unicellular with nonrigid cell wall; variable shapes; free living (needs no host to survive)	• Contact • Airborne • Common vehicle	• *Mycoplasma pneumoniae* (commonly causes primary atypical pneumonia) • *Mycoplasma hominis* (commonly causes nongonococcal urethritis)
Fungi Two main types: molds (multicellular, tubular shape) and yeasts (unicellular, round, or oval shaped); free living (needs no host to survive)	• Contact • Common vehicle • Vector	• *Aspergillus fumigatus* (commonly causes ear, nose, and lung infections) • *Penicillium chrysogenum* (used in penicillin production) • *Candida albicans* (causes vaginitis)
Rickettsia Unicellular with rigid cell wall; rod or oval shaped; needs host to survive.	• Vector	• *Rickettsia prowazekii* (causes epidemic typhus) • *Rickettsia rickettsii* (causes Rocky Mountain spotted fever)
Protozoa	• Contact (direct	• *Trichomonas vaginalis*

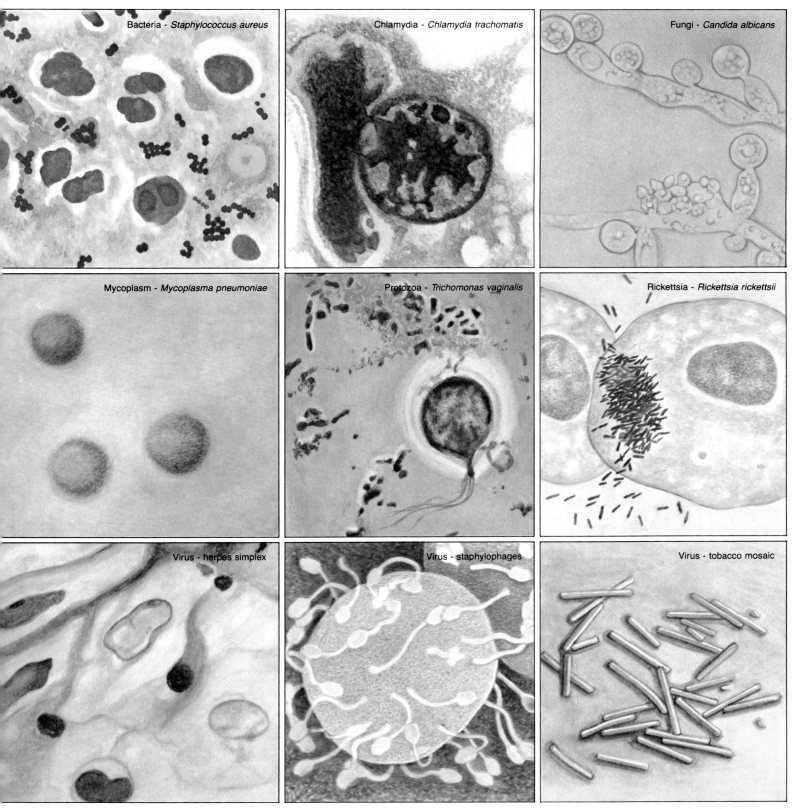

These illustrations have been tinted to enhance the detail. Adapted from microscopic photos, Abbott Laboratories.

Microbiology

Common microorganisms found in humans

Microorganism. What comes to mind when you hear that word? If you're like most nurses, you probably think of infection. But microorganisms aren't always harmful. A normally functioning body depends on microorganisms. However, microorganisms harmless in one part of the body can cause infection in another.

Use this illustration as a guide to the body's normal microorganisms.

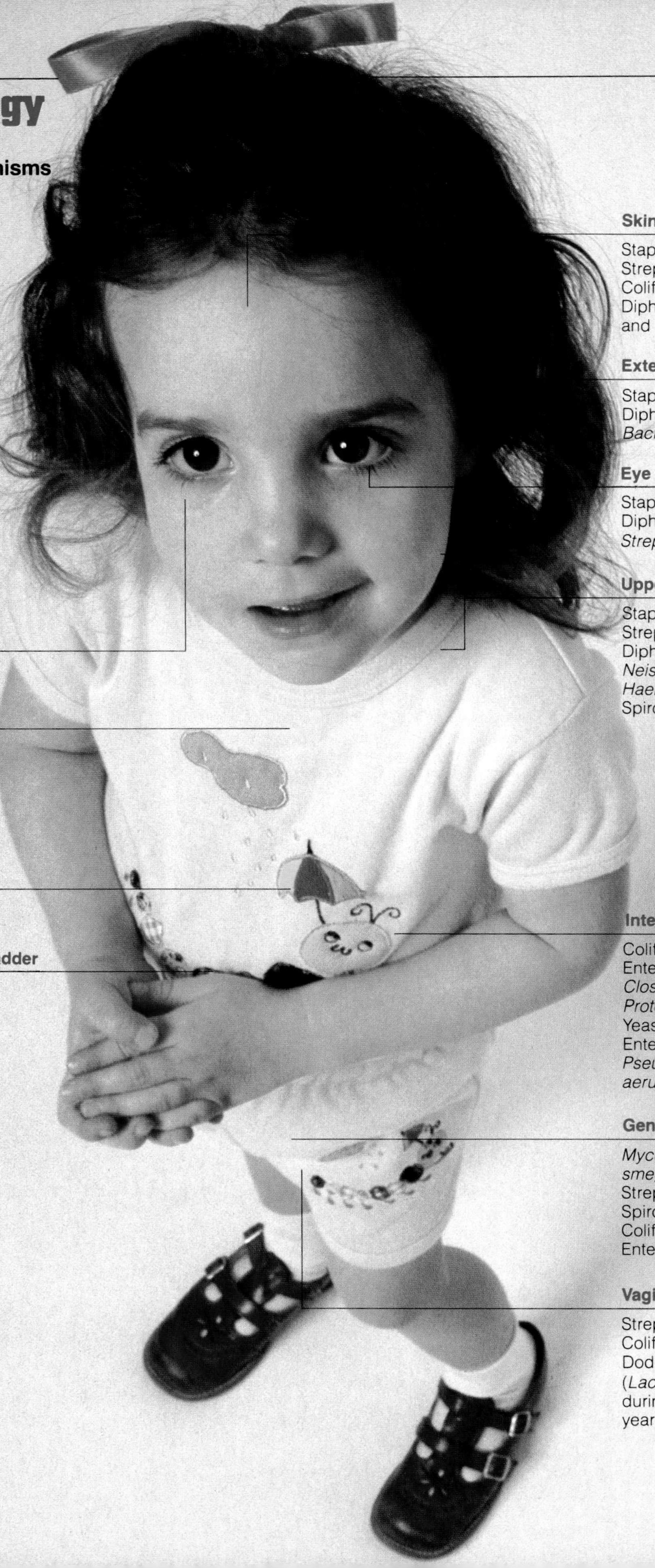

Sinuses

Essentially sterile

Trachea/bronchi/lungs

Essentially sterile

Stomach

Essentially sterile

Kidneys, ureters, and bladder

Essentially sterile

Skin

Staphylococci	*Proteus* species
Streptococci	*Pseudomonas* species
Coliforms	*Bacillus* species
Diphtheroids (aerobic and anaerobic)	Fungi (lipophilic)

External ear

Staphylococci	*Gaffkya tetragena*
Diphtheroids	Nonpathogenic acid-fast organisms
Bacillus species	

Eye

Staphylococci	*Streptococcus pneumoniae*
Diphtheroids	
Streptococcus viridans	

Upper respiratory tract

Staphylococci	*Streptococcus pneumoniae*
Streptococci	
Diphtheroids	Certain amoebas
Neisseria species	Actinomycetes
Haemophilus species	*Candida albicans* and other fungi
Spirochetes	

Intestinal tract

Coliforms	*Penicillium* species
Enterococci	Aerobic and anaerobic streptococci
Clostridium species	
Proteus species	Staphylococci
Yeasts	*Alcaligenes faecalis*
Enteroviruses	*Bacteroides* species
Pseudomonas aeruginosa	Lactobacilli

Genital tract (urethra)

Mycobacterium smegmatis	Lactobacilli
	Mycoplasmas
Streptococci	*Proteus* species
Spirochetes	Staphylococci
Coliforms	Diphtheroids
Enterococci	Saprophytic yeasts

Vagina

Streptococci	Diphtheroids
Coliforms	*Candida albicans*
Doderlein's bacilli (*Lactobacillus* species) during childbearing years	*Staphylococcus aureus* (normal for approximately 10% of the female population)

Understanding the chain of infection

You've probably cared for many patients with infections. But, have you ever wondered how infections develop?

The chain of infection consists of three basic links: a microorganism that causes the infection (an agent); a method of transmitting the agent (mode of transmission); and a susceptible organism for the agent to invade (a host). If any of the links are missing, the chain is incomplete and no infection will develop.

Of course, the presence of all three links doesn't always lead to an infection. Other interrelated factors are involved, such as:
• the relationship between agent's dose and its virulence
• the host's response to agent
• the stage of agent's infectiousness.

Agent
The first link in any infection is the agent. For the agent to grow and multiply, it needs a reservoir, such as water or human tissue.

Next, the agent needs a way of leaving the reservoir. In man, this is known as the port of exit. Common ports include the respiratory, gastrointestinal, and genitourinary tracts.

Then the agent needs a way to reach the host.

Mode of transmission
The second link in the infection chain is the agent's mode of transmission. Four modes exist: contact, airborne, common vehicle, and vector.

Chances are you're most familiar with the three types of contact transmission shown above: *direct* (for example, touching the infected site or kissing an infected person—top right); *indirect* (touching an inanimate object contaminated by a patient with an infection—bottom left); and *airborne* (contacting droplets from an infected person who sneezes—middle left).

Breathing in the residue of evaporated sneeze droplets (known as droplet nuclei) is also an example of airborne transmission. As you know, these infected particles can remain suspended in the air for hours or possibly days.

The common vehicle mode also transmits infection through an inanimate object; for example a multidose medicine vial. But, in this mode, the object was contaminated by something other than a person; for example, a dirty needle.

The last transmission mode, *vector,* is less common in a hospital than the other three modes. With this mode, the infection is transmitted by a nonhuman carrier; for example, by an arthropod (middle right).

Host
Once the agent's transmitted to the host, it needs to find a port of entry; for example, through a cut or the host's respiratory tract.

After it enters the body, the agent begins replicating. Then, the body's natural defense mechanisms (such as white blood cells and antibodies) attempt to kill it. But, suppose the host does not have adequate natural defense mechanisms or the agent's extremely virulent. In such a case, the agent continues to replicate. This, combined with the body's response, is *infection.* But remember, you can prevent or control infection by eliminating any link in the chain we've discussed.

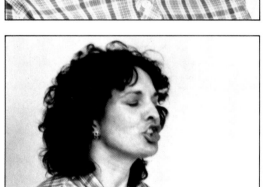

Transmitting host

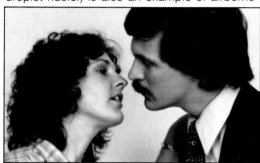

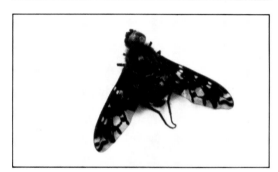

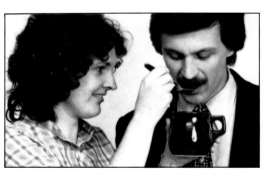

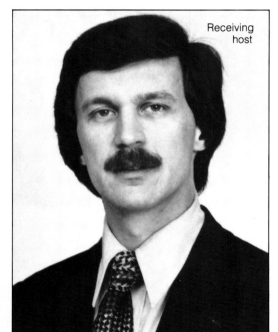

Receiving host

Microbiology

How your body controls infection

Consider the following situation: While breaking open a medication ampule, you cut your finger. Soon after, your finger feels warm and painful. It also appears red and swollen. Wondering why? Here's the reason:

When the skin's broken, as in a finger cut, your body loses its first line of defense, allowing microorganisms to enter through the cut. The redness and swelling result from the body's protective response. Histamine from the injured tissues has caused an increased blood flow to the area, as well as local edema.

Now, let's assume an infection develops. What happens next? Study the following information to refresh your memory.
• Fibrinogen from the edematous fluid forms clots in the tissue spaces around the cut to contain the microorganisms and their toxic products.
• White blood cells begin infiltrating this contained area (top illustration).
• White blood cells surround and destroy each microorganism, then eventually die (middle illustration).
• The accumulation of dead white blood cells, microorganisms, and necrotic tissue forms pus (bottom illustration). As the pus accumulates, an abscess may develop in the area confined by the fibrinogen clots.
• Let's say an abscess develops. It may break open internally or externally (releasing pus); or the contents may be reabsorbed slowly by the body.
• When white blood cells have destroyed all the microorganisms, pus production stops. Then, all the remaining pus is either released or reabsorbed. At this time, tissue granulation begins, and the cut heals.

*Illustrations adapted from photographs by Lennart Nilsson.

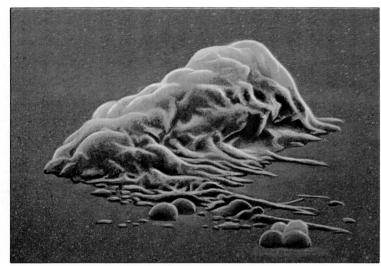

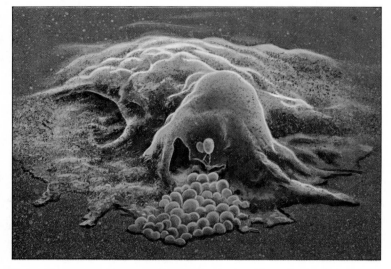

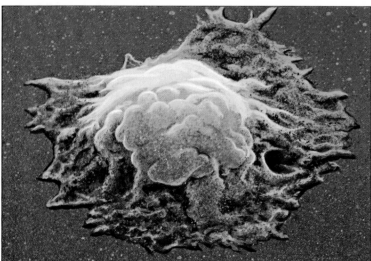

Nosocomial infections

When we talk about a nosocomial infection, we're referring to specific signs and symptoms not present or about to surface when a patient's admitted to the hospital. A nosocomial infection is usually hospital-associated.

Whenever a patient's resistance is lowered, whether from surgery, trauma, or disease, microorganisms in his body may multiply, and an infection may develop. A nosocomial infection can come from organisms that the patient has within his body. These organisms are said to be an endogenous source. Or, the infection may be exogenous, developing from organisms outside his body, within the hospital environment, or from within the community.

As you probably know, a nosocomial infection is most apt to occur wherever a patient's receiving invasive therapy, such as an intravenous line, central venous pressure line, surgical wound, or tracheostomy site. Or, an infection may develop at a trauma site. But, remember, not every patient in these situations will develop a nosocomial infection.

Nosocomial infections may occur in any hospital unit. However, they're more likely to occur in high-risk areas, such as intensive-care units, burn units, or surgical units.

Identifying common nosocomial infections

Type of nosocomial infection	Signs and symptoms	Common causative organisms	Nursing considerations
Skin and vascular system Associated with intravenous (I.V.) therapy	• Puncture-site inflammation, with possible purulent drainage • Inflammation along cannulated vein (phlebitis) • Fever • Signs of generalized sepsis: diaphoresis, shock, nausea, vomiting • Positive specimen culture from I.V. cannula or puncture site	• *Staphylococcus epidermidis* • Enterococci • *Staphylococcus aureus* • *Klebsiella* species • *Pseudomonas aeruginosa* • *Citrobacter freundii* • *Proteus* species • *Candida* species • *Escherichia coli*	• Before administering I.V. solution, check bottle for cracks, leaks, or particles in the solution. If you see any, return the bottle to the pharmacy and obtain a new bottle. (For more information on I.V. administration, see the NURSING PHOTOBOOK MANAGING I.V. THERAPY.) • Maintain aseptic technique when inserting I.V. catheter and changing dressing. • Remember to apply antimicrobial ointment at insertion site, and again with every dressing change. • Securely tape I.V. catheter in place to prevent it from moving in vein. • Routinely replace I.V. bottle, administration set, catheter, and dressing every 24 to 48 hours, or according to your hospital's policy. • Before administering I.V. drugs, clean the injection port thoroughly with alcohol or Betadine, according to your hospital's policy. • If inflammation's present at insertion site, remove the catheter immediately. Then, using sterile scissors, cut the catheter's tip and place it in a sterile culture tube, according to hospital policy. Label tube and send it to the lab immediately for analysis. With sterile equipment, restart the I.V. in a different vein.
Gastrointestinal system Associated with food	• Nausea; vomiting; bloody, mucoid diarrhea • Fever • Positive stool specimen culture	• *Clostridium perfringens* • *Clostridium botulinum* • *Staphylococcus aureus* • Salmonellae • *Escherichia coli* • Shigellae • *Yersinia enterocolitica*	• Obtain stool specimen for culture, as ordered. Label specimen and send it to the lab for analysis. • Follow isolation procedures, as ordered. • Administer antibiotics I.V., as ordered. • Provide adequate fluid intake, orally or I.V., as ordered, to replace lost fluid.
Respiratory system Associated with respiratory therapy (or lack of it)	• Fever • Leukocytosis • Cough with tenacious respiratory secretions • New or progressive pulmonary infiltrate on X-ray • Positive sputum culture	• *Klebsiella* species • *Pseudomonas aeruginosa* • Staphylococci (coagulase-positive) • *Escherichia coli* • *Enterobacter* species • *Streptococcus pneumoniae*	• Obtain sputum specimen for culture, as ordered. Label it and send to lab. • Administer antibiotics, orally or I.V., as ordered. • Provide respiratory therapy (turning, coughing, deep breathing, chest percussions) to help loosen secretions. • Administer oxygen, as ordered. • Make sure respiratory equipment is properly cleaned, disinfected, and maintained. • Urge patient to stop smoking, if applicable.

Microbiology

Identifying common nosocomial infections continued

Type of nosocomial infection	Signs and symptoms	Common causative organisms	Nursing considerations
Genitourinary system Associated with catheters	• Painful, burning sensation around catheter • Cloudy, foul-smelling urine • Back pain • Fever, chills • Possible spasms in bladder and suprapubic areas • Possible blood in urine • Positive urine specimen culture	• *Escherichia coli* • *Proteus* species • Enterococci • *Klebsiella* species • *Pseudomonas* species • *Candida* species	• Use strict aseptic technique when catheterizing patient. • If possible, do not place patients with indwelling (Foley) catheters in the same room, to prevent cross infection. • After the catheter's inserted, tape drainage tubing securely in place to prevent catheter movement in the urethra. Make sure the catheter's securely attached to the drainage tube and urine runs freely into the drainage bag. Always keep drainage bag below the level of your patient's bladder. Empty drainage bag when two thirds full, taking care not to contaminate bag. • Twice each day (or according to your hospital's policy), wash patient's perineal area with Betadine solution or soap and warm water. • Irrigate catheter only if ordered, maintaining strict aseptic technique. Discard irrigating set after each use. • Change indwelling (Foley) catheter when it malfunctions, when an obstruction occurs, or as ordered.
All body systems Associated with surgery	• Swelling, redness, and pain around incision, with purulent, foul-smelling drainage • Fever • Leukocytosis • Positive wound specimen culture	• *Staphylococcus aureus* • *Escherichia coli* • *Pseudomonas aeruginosa* • *Proteus* species • *Bacteroides* species	• Obtain wound culture, as ordered. Label specimen and send to the lab for analysis. • Provide wound and skin isolation, as necessary. • Administer antibiotics, orally or I.V., as ordered. • Maintain aseptic technique when changing dressing and applying antimicrobial medications, as ordered.
All body systems Associated with burns	• Redness, pain, and swelling around burn site, with possible purulent drainage • Odor • Positive culture from burn site specimen • Leukocytosis • Signs of sepsis: diaphoresis, shock, nausea, vomiting	• *Pseudomonas aeruginosa* • *Staphylococcus aureus* • *Escherichia coli* • *Klebsiella* species • *Proteus* species • *Candida* species • *Streptococcus pyogenes* (group A beta-hemolytic)	• If patient has second- and third-degree burns on 10% or more of his body, have him placed in burn unit, and provide strict protective isolation, as ordered. • Obtain cultures of infected burn sites, as ordered. Label and send to lab. • Administer antibiotics, I.V., as ordered. • Maintain aseptic technique when changing dressing and applying antimicrobial medications, as ordered. • To promote healing, provide adequate nutrition (orally, through nasogastric tube, or with total parenteral nutrition). • Be prepared to assist with wound debridement.

Noscomial infections: Prevention and control

Preventing your patient from developing a nosocomial infection is important, but you'll also want to help control infection if it occurs. The tips below will help you prevent or control an infection:
• Always use proper hand-washing technique when caring for your patient.
• Try to keep patients with infections away from other patients.
• If possible, do not care for a recent surgery patient while caring for a patient with an infectious disease.
• Change surgical dressings daily or as ordered, maintaining strict aseptic technique.
• Clean an incision thoroughly and apply antibiotic or antimicrobial ointment, as ordered.

Nurses' guide to common viral diseases

How familiar are you with viral diseases? For example, do you know which virus causes mumps? Or chicken pox? Do you know when to isolate a patient exposed to German measles? If you're unsure, study the following chart. It lists the causes, and signs and symptoms of common viral diseases.

When caring for any patient with a viral disease, you have two main nursing responsibilities:
• Provide symptomatic relief for your patient, because antibiotics don't affect a viral disease.
• Help prevent the spread of disease by always using proper hand-washing technique and taking other preventive measures, such as isolation procedures (as indicated).

RUBELLA
(German measles)
caused by rubella virus

Incubation period
• 14 to 21 days

Period of communicability
• Begins during prodromal period and lasts until rash disappears.
• Lasts for several months in infants.

Signs and symptoms
Prodromal (1 to 5 days)
• Tender swelling of suboccipital, postauricular, and postcervical glands
• Malaise, lymphatic swelling (may not be present in adolescents or adults)
Specific (3 to 4 days)
• Pinkish rash, beginning on face and spreading to trunk and extremities; stiff joints; headache; inflamed nasal mucous membrane; and pruritis
• Occasionally, patient is asymptomatic.

Nursing considerations
• Apply calamine lotion topically to relieve pruritis.
• Administer analgesics and antipyretics, such as aspirin or acetaminophen, orally or rectally, to relieve joint pain and reduce fever, as ordered.
• Take a careful patient admission history. If he was exposed to the virus within 3 weeks before hospital admission, place patient in respiratory isolation.
• Keep newborn infants with congenital rubella in strict isolation, because contagious excretions may continue for several months after birth.
• Isolate contagious patient from women with low rubella titer who are pregnant or in childbearing years.
• If patient's susceptible to viral disease, recommend that he be discharged within 7 days after any exposure. If patient must remain in hospital after the seventh day, place him in respiratory isolation for 2 weeks, as ordered.

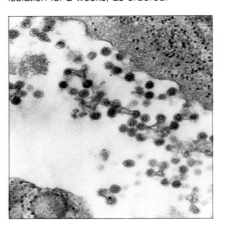

RUBEOLA
(measles)
caused by rubeola virus

Incubation period
• 7 to 14 days

Period of communicability
• Begins 2 to 4 days before rash appears and lasts until rash disappears.

Signs and symptoms
Prodromal (3 to 5 days)
• Fever, cough, profuse nasal discharge, conjunctivitis, and Koplik's spots on buccal mucosa
Specific (3 to 5 days)
• Fever 101° to 104° F. (38.3° to 40° C); pruritis; and maculopapular rash on face 2 to 3 days after Koplik's spots appear. Rash spreads to trunk and extremities within 24 hours.

Nursing considerations
• Keep patient on complete bed rest until fever subsides.
• To reduce fever, administer antipyretics, such as aspirin or acetaminophen, orally or rectally, as ordered.
• Apply calamine lotion topically to relieve pruritis.
• If patient is susceptible to viral disease, recommend that he be discharged within 7 days after any exposure. If patient must remain in hospital after the seventh day, place him in respiratory isolation for 1 week.

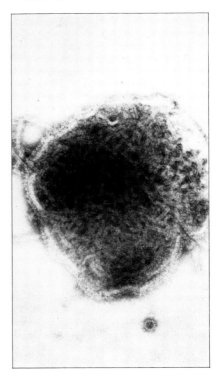

Microbiology

INFECTIOUS MONONUCLEOSIS
caused by Epstein-Barr virus (herpes)

Incubation period
- 14 to 42 days

Period of communicability
- Unknown

Signs and symptoms
Prodromal (5 to 7 days)
- Malaise, fatigue, headache, and chills
Specific (7 to 28 days)
- Fever 101° to 104° F. (38.3° to 40° C.), sore throat, spleen enlargement (on palpation), lymph node swelling and tenderness, and diarrhea

Nursing considerations
- Keep patient on complete bed rest until fever subsides.
- Encourage patient to drink fluids frequently.
- Administer 5% dextrose in water, I.V., as ordered.
- To reduce fever and relieve pain, administer analgesics and antipyretics, such as aspirin, orally, as ordered.
- If fever remains high for 12 to 24 hours after administering aspirin, be prepared to use a hypothermia blanket.
- Provide throat lozenges and saline-solution gargles, as ordered, to relieve sore throat.

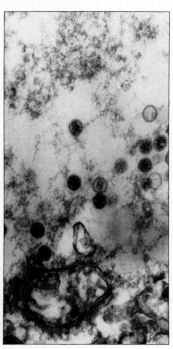

EPIDEMIC PAROTITIS
(mumps)
caused by paramyxovirus

Incubation period
- 12 to 26 days

Period of communicability
- Begins 1 to 6 days before symptoms occur and lasts until swelling disappears.

Signs and symptoms
Prodromal (12 to 14 hours)
- Chills, headache, anorexia, malaise, and fever 100° to 104° F. (37.8° to 40° C.).
Specific (10 to 14 days)
- Initial swelling of one or both parotid glands, later spreading to front of face and behind ears; chewing or swallowing painful

Nursing considerations
- Keep patient on complete bed rest until fever subsides.
- Provide a soft diet to reduce pain from chewing.
- Encourage patient to drink fluids frequently.
- To reduce fever and relieve pain, administer antipyretics and analgesics, such as aspirin, orally or rectally, as ordered.
- Administer phenobarbitol (Luminal*) orally for sedation, as ordered.

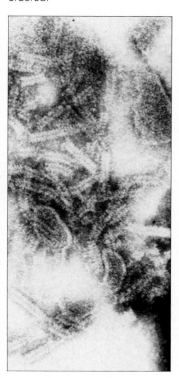

VARICELLA
(chicken pox)
caused by varicella-zoster virus

Incubation period
- 14 to 21 days

Period of communicability
- Begins 1 day before symptoms occur and lasts until lesions become encrusted (about 6 days after vesicles appear).

Signs and symptoms
Prodromal (24 to 36 hours)
- Mild headache, low grade fever 100° to 101° F. (37.8° to 38.3° C.) and malaise
Specific (7 to 14 days)
- Teardrop-shaped vesicles (surrounded by reddened area) on trunk 24 to 36 hours after prodromal symptoms appear. Rash usually spreads to face and arms within 24 hours.
- Pruritis

Nursing considerations
- Apply calamine lotion topically and administer antihistamines, such as diphenhydramine hydrochloride (Benadryl*), as ordered, to relieve pruritis.
- Keep patient in strict isolation until skin lesions become encrusted.
- Keep patients with this virus separated from patients receiving immunosuppressive medication.
- Isolate patient with virus from women with low varicella titer who are pregnant or in child-bearing years.

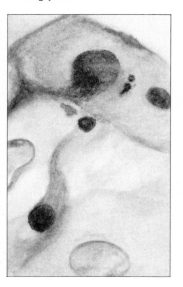

INFLUENZA A
caused by type A influenza virus

INFLUENZA B
caused by type B influenza virus

INFLUENZA C
caused by type C influenza virus

Incubation period
- 1 to 2 days

Period of communicability
- Unknown

Signs and symptoms
Specific (2 to 5 days)
- Fever 102° to 103° F. (38.9° to 39.4° C.), chills, cough, sore throat, generalized aches and pains (especially in the back and legs), mild burning in substernal area, stuffy or runny nose, weakness, headache, anorexia, nausea, vomiting, and diarrhea

Nursing considerations
- Keep patient on complete bed rest until temperature remains normal for 24 to 48 hours.
- Be careful not to contaminate yourself or others when handling respiratory secretions.
- Keep patient with virus away from susceptible patients.
- To reduce fever and relieve pain, administer antipyretics and analgesics, such as aspirin, orally, as ordered.
- Encourage patient to drink fluids frequently.
- Provide throat lozenges or saline-solution gargles, as ordered, to relieve sore throat.

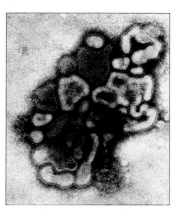

*Available in both the United States and in Canada

Learning about hepatitis

As you know, hepatitis is usually classified into three types: hepatitis A, hepatitis B, and hepatitis non-A, non-B. Each type differs according to the causative virus, the periods of incubation and communicability, and the primary modes of transmission. However, the signs and symptoms of all three types of hepatitis are divided into two stages: the initial or *prodromal* stage, and the later or *specific* stage.

When caring for a patient with hepatitis, taking an accurate history becomes particularly important. Be sure to ask your patient about his living conditions and daily activities (specifically his sexual contacts). This information may provide clues about the infection's source. In addition, you'll want to talk with your patient and his family about the virus. Your patient may be confused or upset about having hepatitis.

To help educate your patient and provide better care, review the following information on each type of hepatitis.

A

HEPATITIS A
Hepatitis A, commonly called infectious hepatitis, is caused by the hepatitis A virus. The signs and symptoms of hepatitis A occur most frequently in children and young adults, although anyone can be affected. Most commonly, it's transmitted through the fecal-oral route. It is also frequently associated with the ingestion of contaminated shellfish.

After a person's exposed to the hepatitis A virus, incubation can last from 14 to 45 days. However, the average period is from 25 to 30 days. A patient can be *infectious* from several weeks before the onset of jaundice to a week or so after its appearance.

The prodromal signs and symptoms of hepatitis A include jaundice, mental and physical fatigue, nausea and vomiting, diarrhea, anorexia, fever, dark urine and light-colored stools, and a moderately enlarged liver, which is tender on palpation. Other signs include increased levels of serum glutamic-oxaloacetic transaminase (SGOT) and serum glutamic-pyruvic transaminase (SGPT). Patients who smoke may also develop a distaste for cigarettes.

After an acute onset, these signs and symptoms can last from 3 to 10 days. The signs and symptoms of type A, on the other hand, usually last from 21 to 42 days. A definite diagnosis is made by the recovery of hepatitis A virus in the blood.

B

HEPATITIS B
Hepatitis B may be more serious than type A. Although its onset is gradual, the virus can become fulminating and possibly chronic. About 10% of all patients with hepatitis B can become permanent carriers of the hepatitis B surface antigen (HB_sAg), sometimes called Australia antigen.

How is the hepatitis B virus spread? Primarily through the parenteral route and through sexual contact, although it may also be associated with I.V. drug use; for example, sharing of needles and other drug paraphernalia. However, as you know, any mucous membrane surface can provide an entry port for the virus. The B virus tends to affect mostly males.

The incubation period for hepatitis B averages 60 to 90 days. But, it can range from 42 to 160 days. Communicability begins with the presence in the blood of hepatitis B surface antigen. However, HB_sAg appears in the blood before the prodromal signs and symptoms appear.

Type B's *specific* signs and symptoms include all those of type A as well as polyarthralgias and rash. As the specific signs and symptoms appear, the HB_sAg level, and consequently infectivity, gradually decreases. A sexual partner has an increased risk of contracting hepatitis B. Prophylaxis (hepatitis B immune globulin), may be indicated in some situations.

NON-A NON-B
AB

HEPATITIS NON-A, NON-B
Hepatitis non-A, non-B, as the name implies, is caused by neither the hepatitis A nor the hepatitis B virus. In fact, diagnosis of this virus is only through exclusion of the other two. The primary mode of transmission is through blood transfusions. Like type B, hepatitis non-A, non-B has an insidious onset. The prodromal and specific signs and symptoms can include any of those found in types A and B. However, no surface antigen is evident. The incubation period ranges from 14 to 180 days, but is usually from 50 to 56 days. The period of communicability is uncertain.

CARE GUIDELINES
When caring for any patient with hepatitis, follow these guidelines:
• Make sure he has adequate bed rest. Complete bed rest is not necessary, unless ordered by the doctor.
• Always wash your hands thoroughly after any contact with your patient or his excretions.
• Follow isolation procedures according to your hospital's policy.
• Allow your patient to eat whatever he can tolerate.

• Administer I.V. fluids, as ordered, if your patient suffers severe nausea and vomiting.
• Instruct your patient to avoid alcoholic beverages during convalescence.
• When having any contact with the blood of a patient with hepatitis type B or non-A, non-B, always wear gloves and use disposable syringes. Label all specimen containers with the word *hepatitis*. Follow your hospital's isolation procedure for collecting and transporting specimens.

Culturing

Let's say the doctor wants to determine why your patient's spiking a temperature after urinary tract surgery. To do this, he may order a blood, urine, or sputum culture. Or, he may order all three of these cultures.

Do you know how to collect a quality specimen for culture? Why postural drainage induces a sputum specimen? What a blood culture x3 is?

For answers to these questions, read the next chapter carefully. In it, you'll find step-by-step procedures and valuable tips for collecting the most common culture specimens.

Rules for obtaining a quality specimen for culture

How familiar are you with culturing? As you probably know, the quality of a specimen affects test validity. To produce reliable results, you must use proper culturing techniques.

Follow these guidelines to ensure quality specimens:
• Explain the procedure to your patient. Try to enlist his full cooperation.
• Wash your hands thoroughly before and after collecting the specimen.
• If possible, don't begin any antibiotic or antimicrobial therapy until after collecting the specimen.
• Use strict aseptic technique.
• Use the appropriate sterile container for the specimen. If you're unsure, check your hospital's procedure manual, or check with the lab.
• Make sure you have a representative specimen of the site. If the site is a large wound or there are multiple infection sites, take specimens from different sites. Use a separate sterile container for each specimen.
• Take a sufficient specimen quantity on the first culture. Repeating the procedure costs time and money, and may cause your patient unnecessary pain. Remember, if the doctor ordered more than one test, obtain a separate specimen for each test.
• Close all specimen containers tightly to prevent spillage and possible contamination. If the container does become soiled, or if the patient's in isolation, wipe it with a bactericide before sending it to the lab.
• Label the specimen container with your patient's name, room number, specimen type, wound location, diagnosis, date, and time collected. Number multiple containers in sequential order. Use an Addressograph® unit to prepare a micro slip for each specimen, or write on the slip by hand. If the patient's on isolation precautions or antibiotic therapy, note this on the micro slip and the culture container.
• Send the specimen to the lab as soon as possible to prevent organism destruction or overgrowth. If transport to the lab is delayed, some specimen types may be refrigerated for a short time. In the case of a viral culture, though, it's best to pack the specimen container in ice and take it to the lab as soon as possible.
• Be sure to document the procedure, date and time in your nurses' notes. This ensures that no one else will repeat the procedure.

How to obtain a nasopharyngeal culture

1 *Does the doctor suspect Bordetella pertussis (whooping cough) in your patient? If so, he'll probably want you to obtain a nasopharyngeal culture. (In some hospitals, the doctor may perform this procedure.) Here's what to do:*

First, gather the necessary equipment: a sterile flexible wire-handled applicator swab (we'll be using a Calgiswab®), a sterile culture medium tube, disposable cup, penlight, and tissues.

Then, explain the procedure to your patient and have him sit at the edge of the bed, facing you. If he's not strong enough to sit upright, place him in high Fowler's position.

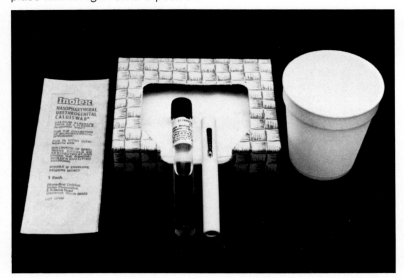

2 Now, instruct your patient to blow his nose, clearing his nasal passages. Then, use the penlight to check his nostrils for patency.

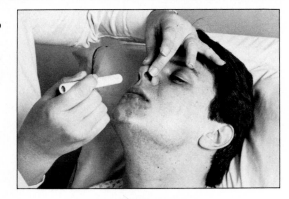

3 Ask your patient to occlude first one nostril, then the other, as he exhales. Note which nostril is more patent.

Next, ask him to cough. Doing so will bring organisms to the nasopharynx, providing a better specimen.

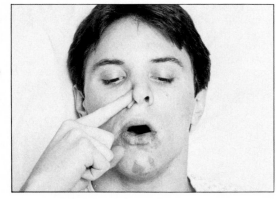

4 Now, loosen the specimen tube cap, as the nurse is doing in this photo. Then, put the tube in the cup.

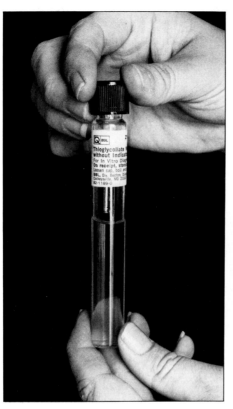

7 When the swab comes in contact with the nasopharynx, gently but quickly rotate it to collect a specimen. *Important:* Be very careful not to perforate the nasopharynx when taking the specimen.
Remove the swab, taking care not to damage the nasal mucous membrane.

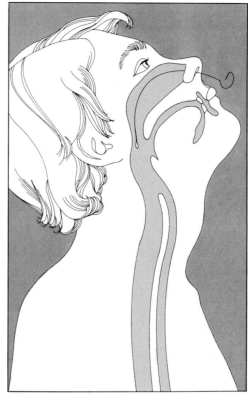

5 Open the package containing the swab. Curve the swab's wire handle to the shape of your patient's nasal passage, as shown here. Avoid contaminating the swab's cotton tip.

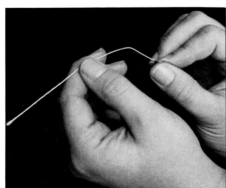

8 Next, remove the cap from the specimen tube, insert the swab, and break off the contaminated end.
Screw the lid onto the specimen tube. Label the tube and send it to the lab with the appropriate lab slip.

6 Ask your patient to tilt his head backward. Then, insert the swab into his more patent nostril.
Advance the swab along the center of the nasal passage until the swab touches your patient's nasopharynx. However, doing so may trigger his cough or gag reflex, so encourage him to relax and breathe through his mouth.

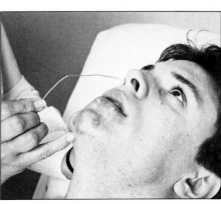
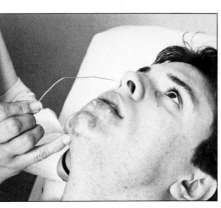

Culturing

Obtaining a throat culture

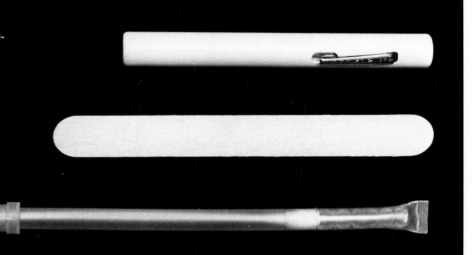

1 *Consider this: 33-year-old Georgia Petrosky comes into the emergency department complaining of a sore throat. After examining Ms. Petrosky, the doctor suspects strep throat. He orders a throat culture to confirm the diagnosis. How do you proceed?*

First, gather the necessary equipment: tongue depressor, penlight, and sterile culture swab with culture medium (we're using a Strep Culturette®).

Then, explain the procedure to Ms. Petrosky. Tell her she'll probably feel some momentary discomfort because her gag reflex may be triggered when you take the specimen. Have her sit on a chair facing you.

Wash your hands.

2 Now, ask Ms. Petrosky to open her mouth and stick out her tongue. Use a tongue depressor to hold down her tongue, as shown.

If your patient starts to gag, remove the tongue depressor and tell her to breathe deeply. Try again when she's relaxed, without placing the tongue depressor as far back in her throat.

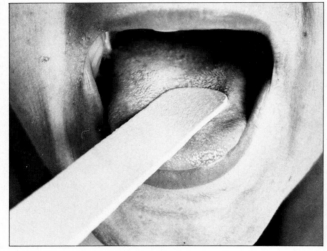

3 Next, shine the penlight into Ms. Petrosky's throat. Note which areas appear inflamed, purulent, or ulcerated.

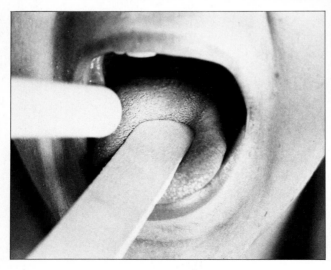

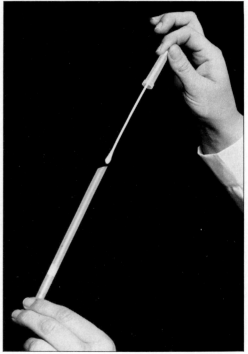

4 Carefully remove the applicator swab from its tube. Be sure the swab doesn't touch the outside of the tube.

Now, ask Ms. Petrosky to open her mouth again. To better see the back of her throat, hold down her tongue with a tongue depressor. This keeps the tongue from touching the swab. Doing so also keeps oral secretions out of the specimen; oral secretions can dilute the specimen or cause an overgrowth of normal mouth microorganisms in the culture.

5 Next, insert the applicator swab into your patient's mouth until it touches the inflamed, purulent, or ulcerated area of her throat. Using a circular motion, firmly and quickly swab the infected area and then remove the swab. Be careful not to touch any other parts of her mouth with the swab.

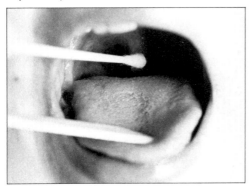

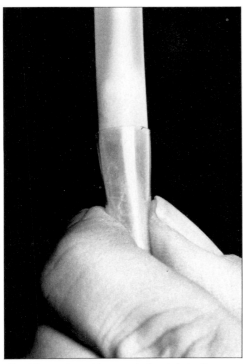

6 Now, place the swab back into the tube. Avoid touching the outside of the tube with the swab.

Crush the ampule of culture medium at the base of the tube, as the nurse is doing here. Then, push the swab into the culture medium. Be sure the swab's completely immersed.

Wash your hands. Then, label the specimen, fill out the appropriate lab slip, and send the specimen to the lab immediately.

Document the procedure in your notes.

Easing sputum collection

Is your patient having trouble coughing up sputum for a specimen? If so, follow these procedures to help loosen his secretions. But, before performing these procedures, check with the doctor to make sure they aren't contraindicated.

Begin by positioning your patient for postural drainage. This allows pulmonary secretions to drain from the lungs into his bronchi or trachea.

What if postural drainage doesn't help your patient? Then, try percussing and vibrating your patient's chest. To percuss, cup each hand and tap alternately on your patient's chest in a firm, rhythmic manner. To vibrate, shake your patient's chest as he slowly exhales. (For further information on postural drainage, percussion, and vibration, see the NURSING PHOTOBOOK PROVIDING RESPIRATORY CARE.)

Suppose your patient still hasn't coughed up sputum. Notify the doctor. He may want the sputum induced through warm aerosol inhalation. To do this, place an aerosol mask attached to a nebulizer over your patient's mouth and nose. Tell your patient to breathe normally. After 15 to 20 minutes, remove the mask and ask your patient to cough.

Note: In some hospitals, a respiratory therapist performs the warm aerosol inhalation procedure. Before beginning, check your hospital's policy.

Collecting a coughed sputum specimen

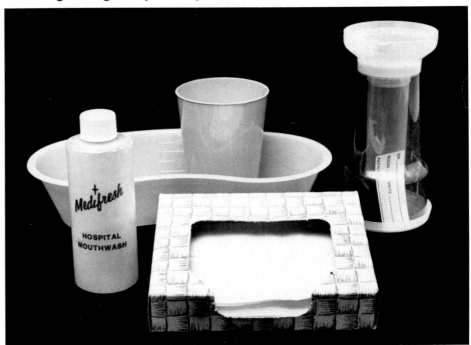

1 *Let's assume Tom DiMarco, a 32-year-old mechanic, has been admitted to your unit with signs of a lower respiratory infection. To confirm the diagnosis, the doctor orders a sputum specimen. As you know, you'll collect the specimen in early morning, having allowed your patient's respiratory secretions to accumulate during the previous night.*

Begin by gathering this equipment: container (in this photostory, the nurse is using a Falcon® sputum collection system); a cup with mouthwash; tissues; and an emesis basin.

Explain to Mr. DiMarco that he'll have to cough deeply and expectorate directly into the container. Demonstrate the proper technique. Be sure he understands that sputum comes from deep within the lungs, unlike saliva, which comes from the mouth.

Note: Remain with your patient during the procedure to ensure a fresh specimen. Never take a specimen from sputum in a bedside container.

Culturing

Collecting a coughed sputum specimen continued

2 Have Mr. DiMarco sit at the edge of the bed. Or, if he's not strong enough, place him in high Fowler's position.
   Instruct him to rinse out his mouth with mouthwash to reduce oral contaminants in the sputum specimen.

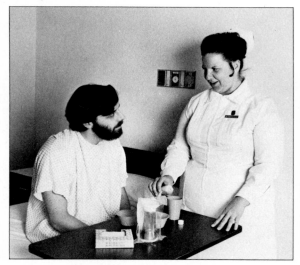

3 Next, hand the opened sputum container to Mr. DiMarco. Tell him to cough the sputum into the container, being careful not to contaminate the outside of the container with the sputum.
   Then, press the lid closed.

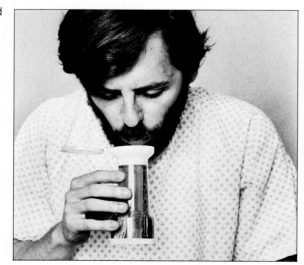

4 Instruct Mr. DiMarco to once again rinse his mouth with mouthwash. Doing so will remove any unpleasant taste in his mouth.

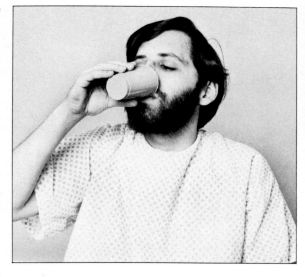

5 Then, holding the container upright, remove the bottom lid. Carefully pull out the specimen tube, the label, and the specimen tube cap, taking care not to spill the collected sputum or contaminate the cap.

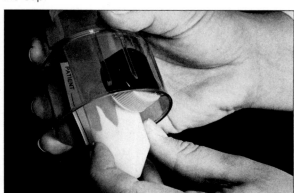

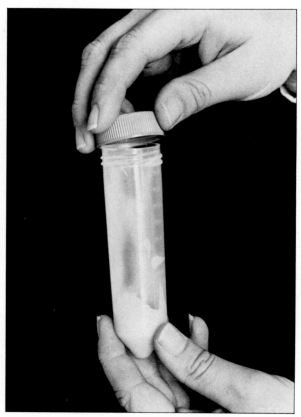

6 Now, screw the cap onto the specimen tube. Label the tube and send it to the lab immediately.
   Important: If the doctor orders a sputum culture x3, collect three separate specimens at three different times during the day or on three consecutive days. Send each specimen to the lab as soon as it's collected. *Never divide a single sputum specimen among three containers.*

Collecting a sputum specimen using nasotracheal suction

1 *Roberta Hancock, a 33-year-old secretary, was admitted to your unit with signs and symptoms of pneumonia (elevated temperature, cough, and chest tenderness on inspiration). She's receiving oxygen via nasal cannula at a rate of 3 liters per minute. The doctor orders a sputum specimen for culture and sensitivity. Because Ms. Hancock can't produce a coughed specimen, you'll need to suction her nasally. Do you know how to collect a sputum specimen using this method? If not, read this photostory.*

First, gather the necessary equipment: sterile suction kit; sputum trap; and tissues. We're using a Regu-Vac® suction kit, which contains a glove, 4 oz. (120 ml) sterile water, a suction catheter and cup; and a Chesebrough-Pond's specimen trap. If your patient's room doesn't have a wall suction unit, you'll also need a portable suction machine.

Note: Before proceeding, check the suctioning machine to be sure it's functioning properly.

Next, explain the procedure to your patient. Tell her it may be briefly uncomfortable, but not painful. Then, place her in either a high or semi-Fowler's position.

Now, wash your hands thoroughly. Using aseptic technique, open the sterile suction kit and the specimen trap. Put on the sterile glove.

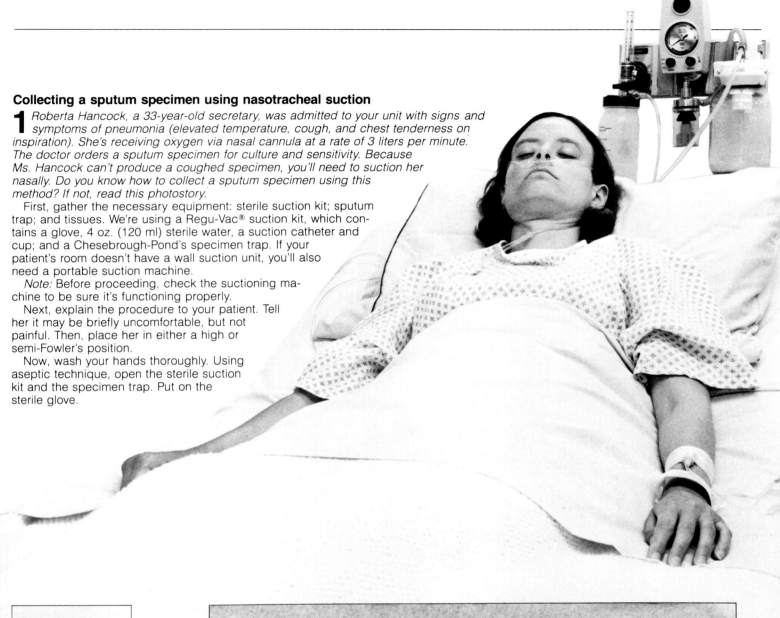

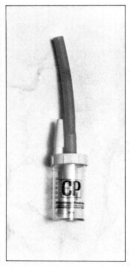

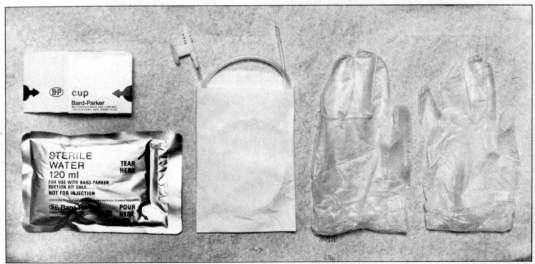

Culturing

Collecting a sputum specimen using nasotracheal suction continued

2 With your gloved hand, squeeze open the kit's cup. Holding the premeasured package of sterile water in your ungloved hand, tear open the package with your gloved hand.
  Pour the sterile water into the cup. Discard the empty package.

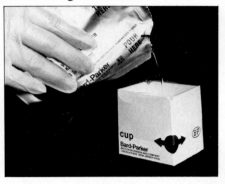

3 Now, with the trap in your gloved hand and the suction machine's tubing in your ungloved hand, insert the trap's rigid connector into the suction tubing. Then grasp the trap's latex tubing with your ungloved hand.

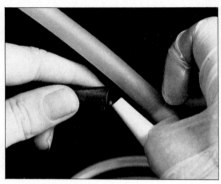

4 With your gloved hand, insert the suction catheter's distal end into the trap's latex tube. Be careful not to contaminate the catheter with your ungloved hand.

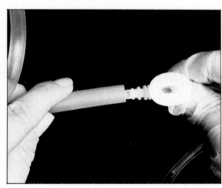

5 Adjust the suction machine so it is set for constant low suction. Then, turn on the machine.

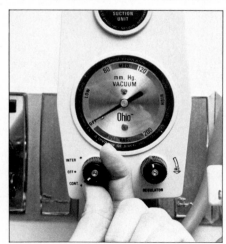

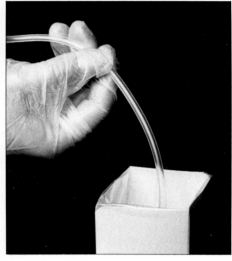

6 Lubricate the tip of the suction catheter by dipping it into the sterile water.
  Caution: Don't place your finger over the suction catheter's valve. Doing so will cause sterile water to enter the trap, interfering with the specimen.
  Now, instruct your patient to take several deep breaths. Remove the nasal cannula.

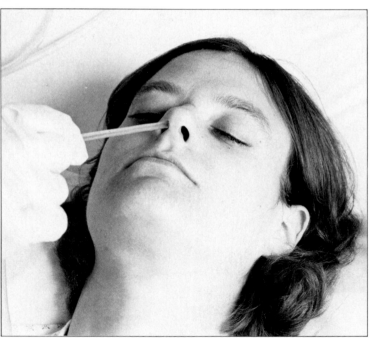

7 Tell your patient to tilt her head back slightly. Gently insert the suction catheter into Ms. Hancock's nostril, using your gloved hand.
  Nursing tip: To make insertion easier, ask your patient to take several deep breaths through her mouth.
  Then, carefully advance the catheter into your patient's trachea. Don't force it. If you meet resistance while advancing the catheter, withdraw the catheter and discard it. Obtain another sterile suction catheter and sterile glove. Repeat the procedure, inserting the catheter into Ms. Hancock's other nostril. Suppose you still meet resistance. Withdraw the catheter and notify the doctor.
  Remember: Don't place your finger over the suction catheter's valve during insertion. Doing so will irritate the mucosa.
  When the catheter's into Ms. Hancock's trachea, withdraw it about ½" (1.3 cm) to prevent damage to the tracheal mucosa.

8 Now, begin suctioning the tracheal secretions into the specimen trap bottle. To do this, intermittently cover the catheter's valve with your gloved thumb (see photo). As you do, slowly withdraw the catheter.

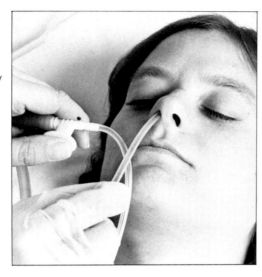

9 When you're finished, use your ungloved hand to give your patient a tissue to blow her nose. With the same hand, turn off the suction machine. Disconnect the suction tubing from the trap's rigid connector.

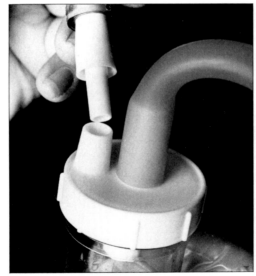

10 Next, disconnect the suction catheter from the trap's latex tubing. Place the specimen trap on the table in an upright position.

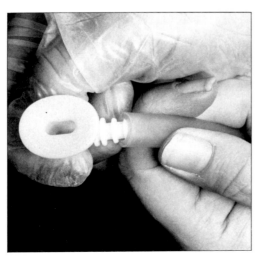

11 Then use your ungloved hand to pull the glove inside out and over the suction catheter, as shown here. Discard both the glove and the catheter into the wastebasket. *Caution:* Avoid touching either the outside of the glove or the catheter with your ungloved hand.

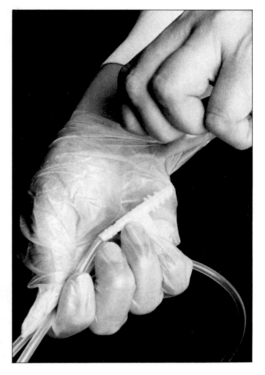

12 Push the latex tubing over the rigid connector, taking care to hold the trap upright. Label the specimen and appropriate lab slip with the patient's name, room number, type of specimen, and the date and time of collection. Send the specimen to the lab as soon as possible (within 30 minutes). *Important:* Do not refrigerate the specimen.

Document the procedure in your nurses' notes.

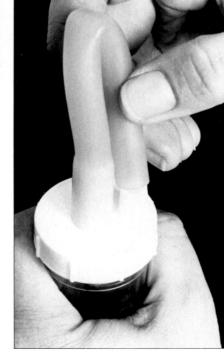

Culturing

Obtaining a cerebrospinal fluid culture

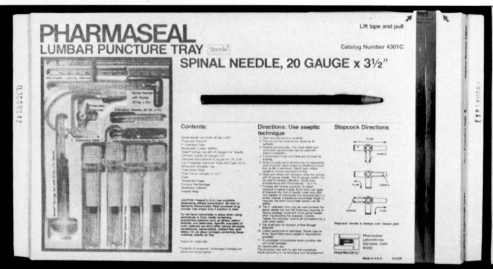
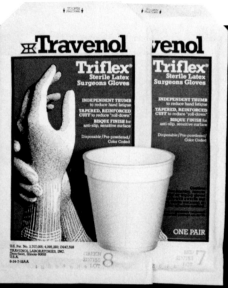

1 *Consider this situation: Your patient's showing signs of meningeal irritation, such as headache, dizziness, and restlessness. To rule out meningitis, the doctor decides to perform a lumbar puncture to obtain cerebrospinal fluid for culture. He asks you to assist. Here's how:*

Begin by gathering the necessary equipment: sterile lumbar puncture tray, two pairs of sterile gloves, grease or wax pencil,

paper cup, and a face mask for the doctor (optional).

Then, thoroughly explain the procedure to your patient and answer any questions he may have. Tell him he'll probably feel pressure during the procedure but it'll last only a few minutes. Reassure him that the doctor will anesthetize the site before he performs the puncture.

Make sure your patient has emptied his bowel and bladder.

2 Now, have your patient lie on his side and bring his knees up toward his chin. Tell him to tuck his head, as shown here. Make sure his spine's curved and his back's at the edge of the bed, close to the doctor. This position opens the spaces between the vertebrae, allowing the doctor to insert the spinal needle more easily. Instruct your patient not to move or twist his spine during the procedure.

Note: Some doctors may prefer the patient to be positioned somewhat differently.

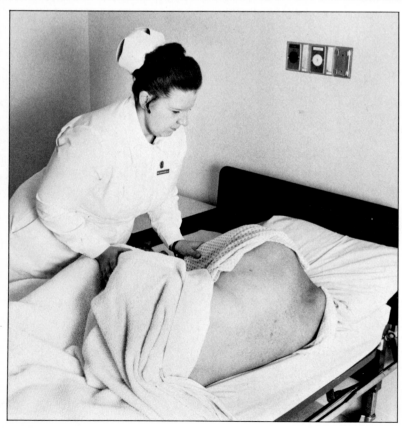

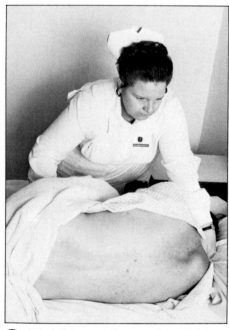

3 What if your patient can't hold this knee/chest position for some reason? Then, place one hand behind his neck and the other behind his knees, as shown here, and pull gently. Help the patient hold this position throughout the procedure.

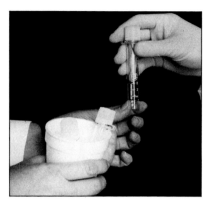

4 The doctor will now begin the procedure, filling several tubes with cerebrospinal fluid. As he does, continue to reassure your patient.

After the doctor fills the first tube, he may hand you the capped tube. Keeping the tube upright, use a grease pencil to mark it No. 1 (unless it's been previously numbered). Then, place the tube in the paper cup.

Repeat this procedure with each tube, numbering them sequentially.

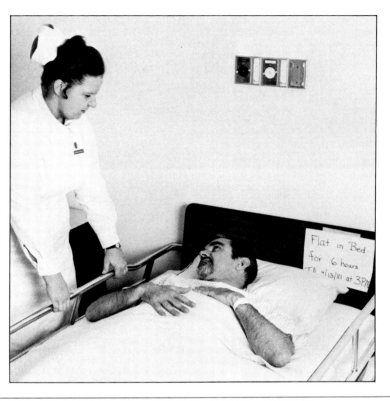

5 When the procedure's completed, place your patient flat on his back. Explain that he will remain in this position 4 to 6 hours, or as ordered. Doing so may help prevent him from getting a spinal headache from spinal fluid loss.

Note: Encourage your patient to drink plenty of fluids to help his body replace lost spinal fluid.

Then, complete the necessary lab slips. If you're sending more than one slip, number them sequentially. Attach the slips to the specimen tubes and send the specimens to the lab immediately. *Never refrigerate them.*

Finally, document the procedure in your notes, including the color, consistency, and amount of spinal fluid removed, the patient's vital signs, and his tolerance of the procedure.

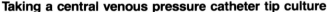

Taking a central venous pressure catheter tip culture

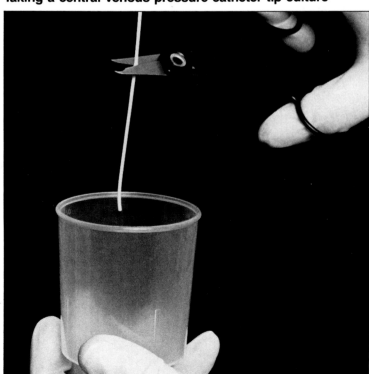

Let's assume your patient's showing signs of infection. The doctor suspects the cause of the infection is your patient's central venous pressure (CVP) catheter. He orders the CVP catheter removed and the tip sent to the lab for culture.

If taking a CVP catheter for culture is a nursing responsibility in your hospital, you'll probably use one of three types of sterile specimen containers: an empty sterile container with a lid, a test tube containing normal saline solution, or a test tube containing a cotton ball saturated with sodium polyanethol sulfonate (SPS). Of the three, the test tube with SPS usually is the best transport medium. Why? The saturated cotton ball provides the correct moisture content without diluting the specimen or letting it dry out.

But, no matter which type you use, the procedure for taking the culture's the same. Once you've removed your patient's dressing and sutures, clean the site with a povidone-iodine (Betadine) wipe, using strict aseptic technique. Then , withdraw the catheter and hold it directly over the container. Cut 2″ to 3″ (5.1 to 7.6 cm) from the tip of the catheter, taking care that it falls into the container.

Note: In some hospitals, the tip's cut off and discarded. Only the section of catheter that was under the skin (about 2″, or 5.1 cm) is sent to the lab.

After capping the container, label and send it directly to the lab with the appropriate slip. (For more details on removing a CVP catheter, see the NURSING PHOTOBOOK MANAGING I.V. THERAPY.)

Suppose the doctor also suspects contaminated I.V. fluid as the infection source. Then, you may also need to send 20 ml of the fluid to the lab, according to your hospital's policy.

Remember to document the procedure, the site's appearance and drainage, and your patient's tolerance for the procedure.

Culturing

Collecting a blood culture

1 *Consider this situation: The doctor suspects septicemia in 43-year-old Donna Ridgeway and orders a blood culture x3. In your hospital, this is a nursing responsibility requiring that three individual blood specimens from different collection sites be timed to precede three different temperature spikes. You'll want to collect the specimens when bacteria is present in the blood.*

Note: As you probably know, the presence of bacteria may be intermittent and may precede, by an hour or more, the onset of fever, chills, and other septicemic signs.

However, in some hospitals the x3 order may mean taking blood specimens on 3 consecutive days or at three specified times during the day, according to doctor's orders. Follow these steps when taking a blood culture:

Explain the procedure to Ms. Ridgeway. Instruct her to notify you when she feels feverish, chilled, or has any other signs indicating a temperature elevation.

Closely monitor and document details of your patient's condition. Then, as Ms. Ridgeway's temperature spikes, prepare to take the blood culture. To do this, gather the necessary equipment: a Vacutainer® blood culture medium tube, Vacutainer sterile needle and sleeve, alcohol and povidone-iodine scrubs or wipes, sterile 3"x3" dry sponges, a tourniquet, and sterile gloves (optional).

Note: Several other acceptable methods exist for obtaining blood cultures. Follow your hospital's policy.

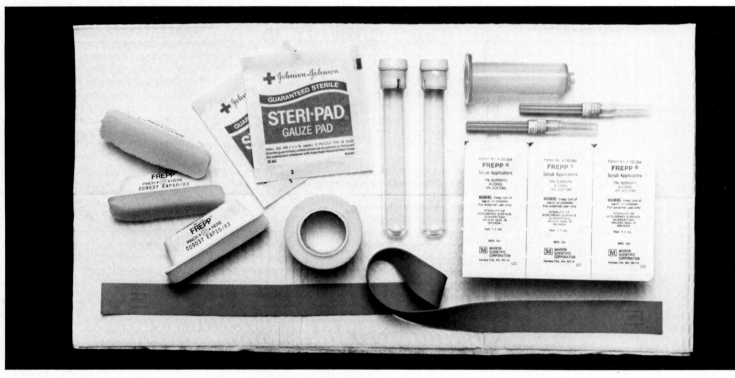

2 Now, wash your hands. Thoroughly clean the top of the medium tube using povidone-iodine and then alcohol.

Next, screw the Vacutainer needle into the sleeve, as the nurse is doing here.

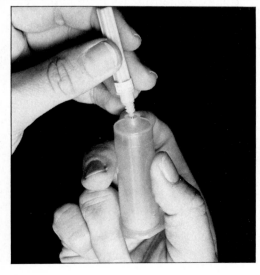

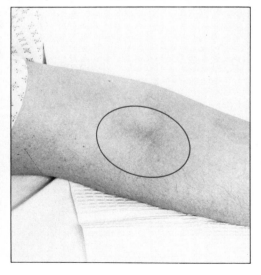

3 Choose the vein from which the specimen is to be drawn. (In this photostory, the nurse will use a vein in the antecubital fossa.) *Remember:* Each time you take a blood specimen, choose a different venipuncture site, to help ensure a quality bacterial-seeded specimen. As you know, bacterial seeding occurs at different times at different sites.

4 Using a circular motion, clean the antecubital fossa with povidone-iodine and then alcohol, beginning at the puncture site and working outward. Discard the wipes.

Repeat this procedure two more times. Pat the area dry with a sterile gauze pad.

Thorough cleaning not only prevents skin organisms from contaminating the specimen, but also prevents additional bacteria from entering the bloodstream. Now tighten the tourniquet.

Important: If you must touch the site again for any reason, put on sterile gloves.

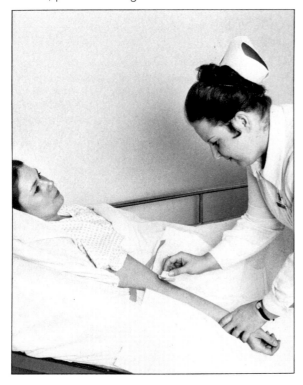

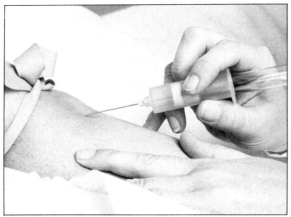

5 Remove the needle cover. Then, with the bevel up, insert the needle into your patient's vein at a 45° angle.

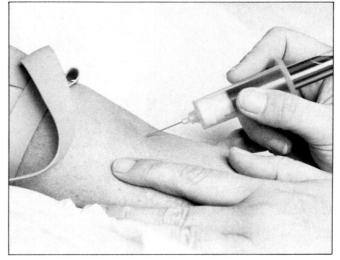
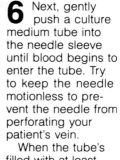

6 Next, gently push a culture medium tube into the needle sleeve until blood begins to enter the tube. Try to keep the needle motionless to prevent the needle from perforating your patient's vein.

When the tube's filled with at least 9 cc of blood, carefully remove it.

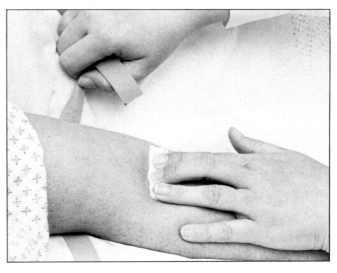

7 Remove the tourniquet from Ms. Ridgeway's arm. Then, as you withdraw the needle, use a dry sponge to apply direct pressure to the puncture site.

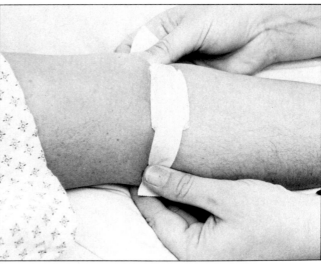

8 After 2 to 3 minutes, remove the sponge and cover the site with a pressure dressing.

Label and send the specimen to the lab immediately.

Document the procedure in your nurses' notes.

Culturing

Collecting a urine specimen for culture

To properly prepare your patient for a urine specimen, have him drink one or two glasses of fluid (unless contraindicated) 30 minutes before the procedure. This will ensure an adequate urine flow.

If your patient has an indwelling catheter or is nonambulatory, you'll need to assist him in obtaining the specimen. But, in most cases, you'll teach your patient how to collect the urine specimen himself. So, give him a copy of one of the home care aids on pages 32-33, and 34. As you discuss the home care aid with him, stress the steps that minimize the risk of contamination.

Give your patient a clean-catch urine kit, and ask him if he has any questions about the specimen collection. Make sure he understands the technique.

After your patient returns the filled cup, or you obtain the urine specimen, label and send it to the lab immediately. If this isn't possible, refrigerate the specimen until you can send it, but be sure it reaches the lab within 6 hours.

Collecting a urine specimen: Closed urinary drainage system

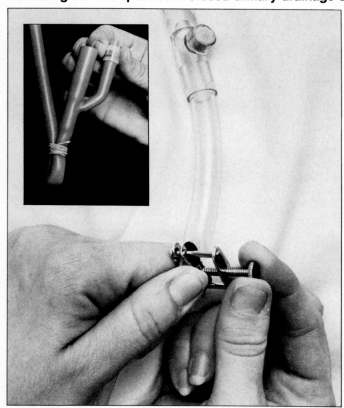

1 *Put yourself in this situation: 64-year-old Ben Snyder, a patient with an indwelling (Foley) catheter, has a suspected urinary tract infection. The doctor orders a urine culture. Here's how to proceed:*

To ensure a sufficient amount of urine, you'll need to block the flow into the drainage bag for 20 to 30 minutes. To do this, clamp the drainage tubing below the aspiration port, as shown here.

[Inset] If your patient's drainage tubing has no aspiration port, clamp the catheter above the Y junction using a rubber band, as shown here.

▣ *Nursing tip:* Put a sign above your patient's bed stating that you've clamped the tubing. Include the time.

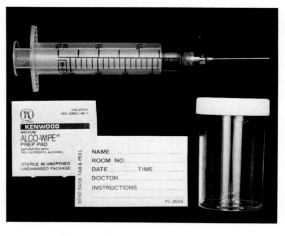

2 When sufficient urine's accumulated, prepare to collect the specimen. Obtain an alcohol or povidone-iodine (Betadine) wipe; a sterile 5 cc syringe and 20G needle; and a sterile plastic specimen container.

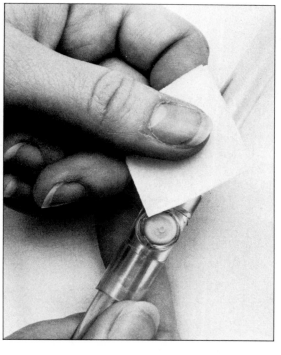

3 Wash your hands. Then, using the wipe, thoroughly clean the aspiration port with a brisk, rubbing motion (creating friction).

4 Expel the air in the syringe. Then, puncture the aspiration port with the needle, as shown here. Aspirate 2 to 5 ml urine.

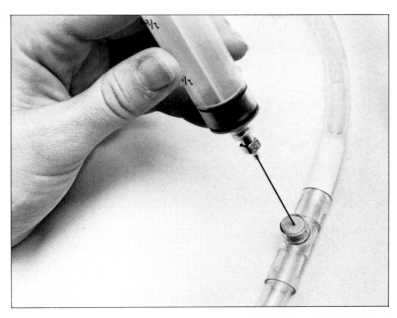

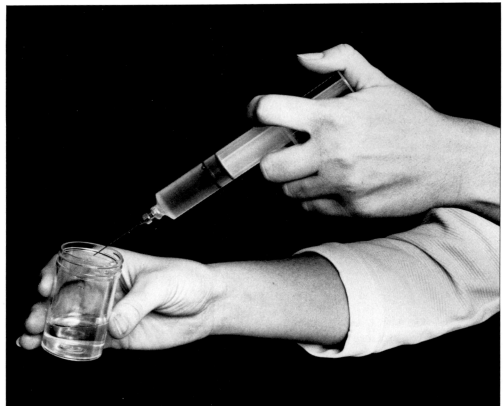

5 Next, withdraw the needle from the port and expel the urine into the sterile specimen container.

Important: When you've finished, remove the clamp or rubber band from the drainage tubing so the urine will flow freely. Also,

discard the sign you placed above your patient's bed.

Put the lid on the specimen container. Label and send the specimen to the lab with the appropriate lab slip.

Remember to document the procedure.

SPECIAL CONSIDERATIONS

Collecting a urine specimen from a nonambulatory patient

Let's say the doctor orders a urine culture for a patient who's on complete bed rest. You'll need to assist your patient in obtaining the specimen. Here's how:

First, make sure your patient's adequately hydrated before collecting the specimen, unless contraindicated.

Then, to prepare for the procedure, place the following opened equipment on an overbed table: midstream urine collection kit (containing a sterile specimen container with lid, three disposable wipes, and a label), washcloth, towel, and soap and water. Help your patient onto a bedpan and put on clean gloves.

Now, follow these steps to take the urine specimen:
• Using a washcloth, clean your patient's perineal area with soap and water.
• Clean the urethral area (as described on pages 32 and 33) using all three disposable wipes. If your male patient's uncircumcised, first retract his foreskin.
• For a female patient, separate her labia with your thumb and index finger, exposing the urinary meatus.
• Ask your patient to begin urinating into the bedpan. After the initial stream, collect a midstream specimen in the sterile urine container. Avoid touching your patient's body with the container.
• When the container's two thirds full, remove it. Tell your patient to finish urinating in the bedpan.
• Dry the urethral area and remove the bedpan. If your patient is an uncircumcised male, ease his foreskin back over the glans.
• Wash your hands.
• Label and send the specimen to the lab with an appropriate lab slip.
• Document the procedure in your nurses' notes. Also, note on your patient's intake and output record the total amount of urine collected. Be sure to include the urine in the specimen container.

Culturing

Self-care

Collecting a urine specimen (for the female patient)

1 Dear Patient:
The doctor suspects you have a urinary tract infection. To confirm his diagnosis, he wants a specimen of your urine so it can be analyzed by the lab.

Carefully follow these instructions for collecting a urine specimen. Doing so will keep outside germs from contaminating the specimen.

First, make sure you have a clean washcloth, towel, soap, water, and a clean-catch urine kit (which the nurse will give you). Remove your clothes from the waist down.

2 Wash your hands thoroughly. Then, using the washcloth, wash your genital area with soap and water. Rinse the area thoroughly and dry it with a towel.

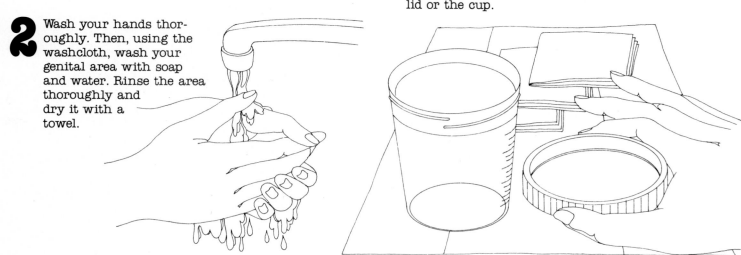

3 Next, place a clean paper towel on a nearby dry surface. Open the three disposable wipes from the clean-catch urine kit and place them on the paper towel.

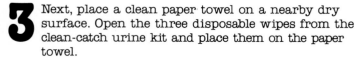
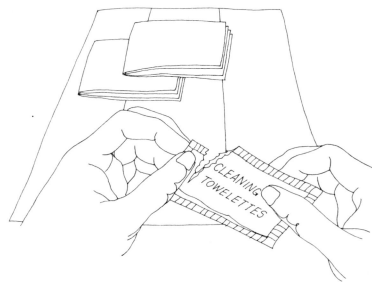

4 Remove the lid from the specimen cup. Place both the cup and the lid (flat side down) next to the wipes. Make sure you don't touch the inside of the lid or the cup.

5 Sit as far back on the toilet as possible. Spread your legs apart.

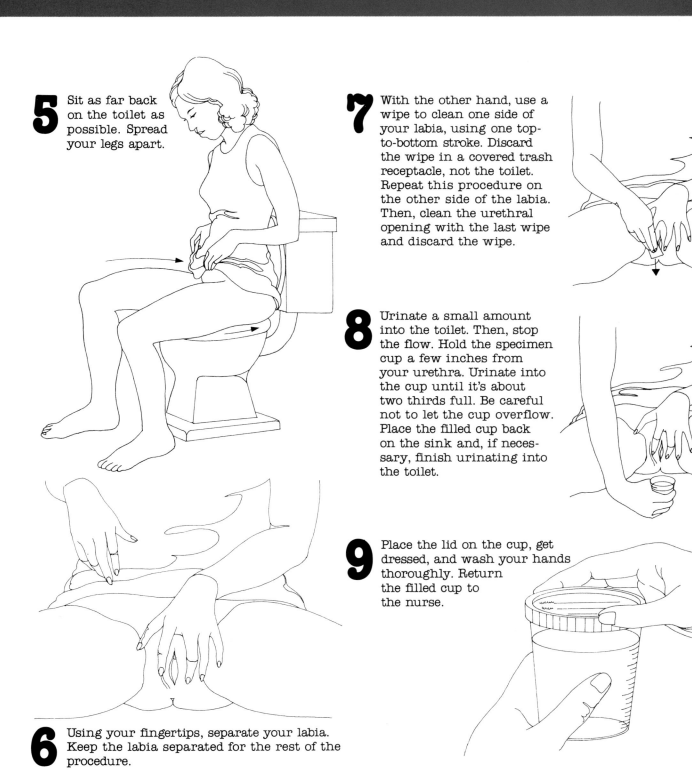

6 Using your fingertips, separate your labia. Keep the labia separated for the rest of the procedure.

7 With the other hand, use a wipe to clean one side of your labia, using one top-to-bottom stroke. Discard the wipe in a covered trash receptacle, not the toilet. Repeat this procedure on the other side of the labia. Then, clean the urethral opening with the last wipe and discard the wipe.

8 Urinate a small amount into the toilet. Then, stop the flow. Hold the specimen cup a few inches from your urethra. Urinate into the cup until it's about two thirds full. Be careful not to let the cup overflow. Place the filled cup back on the sink and, if necessary, finish urinating into the toilet.

9 Place the lid on the cup, get dressed, and wash your hands thoroughly. Return the filled cup to the nurse.

Culturing

Self-care

Collecting a urine specimen (for the male patient)

1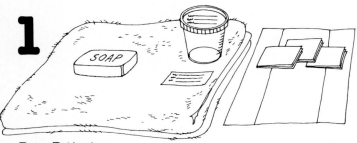

Dear Patient:

The doctor suspects you have a urinary tract infection. To confirm his diagnosis, he wants a specimen of your urine cultured and analyzed by the lab.

Carefully follow these instructions for collecting a urine specimen. Doing so will keep you from contaminating it.

First, make sure you have a clean towel, soap, water, and a clean-catch urine kit (which the nurse will give you).

Wash your hands thoroughly. Place a clean paper towel on a nearby dry surface. Then, open the three disposable wipes and place them on the paper towel.

2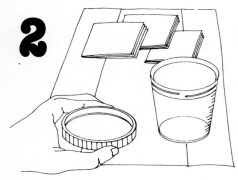

Remove the lid from the specimen cup. Place both the cup and the lid (flat side down) next to the wipes. Make sure you don't touch the inside of the lid or the cup.

3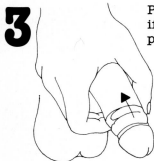

Prepare to urinate. (However, if you're uncircumcised, first pull back your foreskin.)

4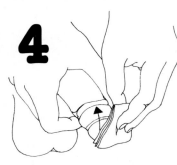

Using a wipe, clean the head of your penis. Clean from the urethral opening toward you, as shown. Then, discard the wipe in a covered trash receptacle, not the toilet. Repeat this procedure with the other wipes.

5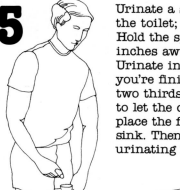

Urinate a small amount into the toilet; then, stop the flow. Hold the specimen cup a few inches away from your penis. Urinate into the cup until you're finished or the cup's two thirds full. Be careful not to let the cup overflow. Replace the filled cup on the sink. Then, if necessary, finish urinating into the toilet.

6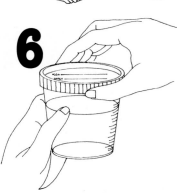

Put the lid on the cup. Remember to wash your hands thoroughly. Then, return the cup to the nurse.

Collecting a urine specimen using straight catheterization (for the female patient)

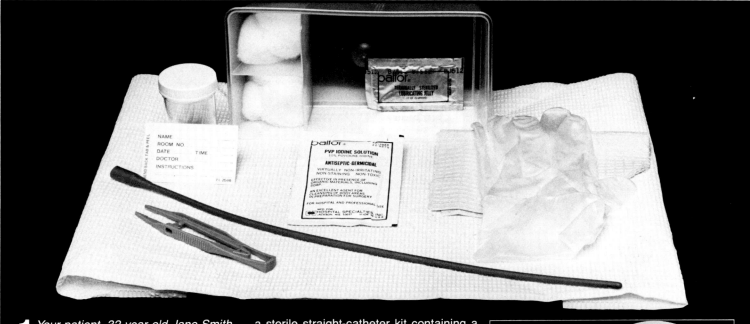

1 *Your patient, 32-year-old Jane Smith, has a postpartum urinary tract infection. The doctor orders a catheter-collected urine specimen for culture and sensitivity testing. To obtain the specimen by straight catheterization, follow these steps:*

Before you begin, check the doctor's orders for catheter size (most straight-catheter kits contain a No. 12 French latex Robinson catheter).

Then, gather the following equipment:
a sterile straight-catheter kit containing a straight catheter, a specimen container, lubricant, cotton balls, povidone-iodine (Betadine) solution, forceps, gloves, and sterile drapes. You'll also need clean gloves; two bed-saver pads; washcloth; towel; soap; and a basin with warm water (see inset). Additionally, obtain a goose-neck lamp to provide direct lighting.

Now, explain the procedure to Ms. Smith. Provide privacy by closing her bed curtain.

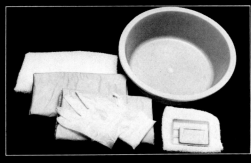

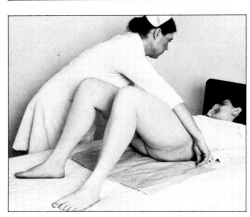

2 Wash your hands. Then, place Ms. Smith flat on her back (if possible) with her knees bent and hips adducted. Slip a bed-saver pad under her buttocks. Then, place her feet 24″ (61 cm) apart. *Note:* If your patient can't lie on her back, position her on her side.

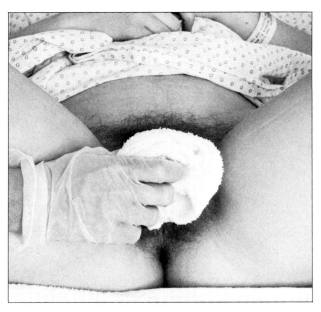

3 Put on the clean gloves. Then, using the wash-cloth, clean your patient's perineum with warm water and soap. Pat the area dry with a towel.

Replace the wet bed-saver pad with a dry pad, remove your gloves, and wash your hands.

Now, place the catheter kit between Ms. Smith's legs (or behind them if she's in a side-lying position).

Using aseptic technique, open the kit. If the catheter's packaged separately, carefully open the package and drop the catheter into the open kit.

Then, maintaining aseptic technique, put on the sterile gloves.

Culturing

Collecting a urine specimen using straight catheterization (for the female patient) continued

4 Now, create a sterile field by placing a sterile drape between Ms. Smith's legs and under her hips. Begin by picking the sterile plastic-coated drape and folding it over your hands, as shown. This prevents contaminating your gloved hands.

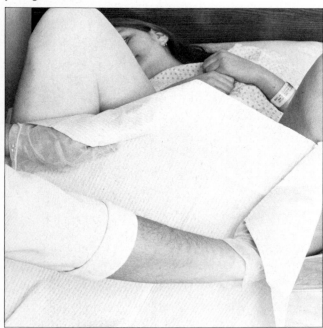

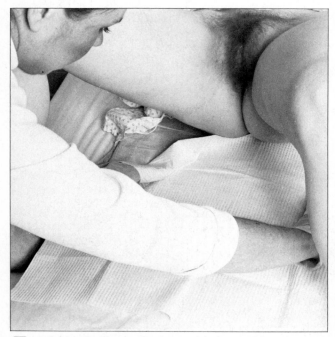

5 Ask Ms. Smith to raise her pelvis by pushing down with her feet. Slide the drape under her buttocks, as the nurse is doing in this photo. Avoid touching her buttocks with your gloved hands. Then, withdraw your hands, and tell her to lower her pelvis onto the drape.

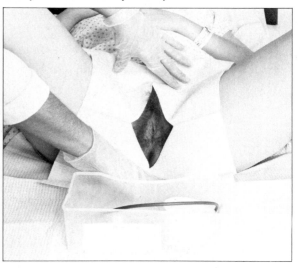

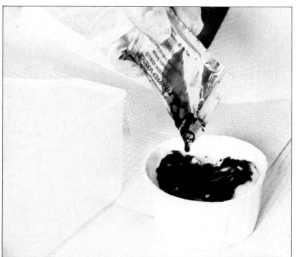

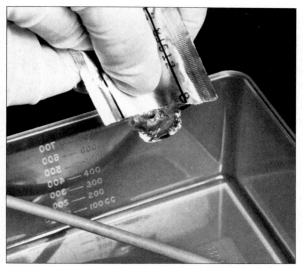

6 Now, position the precut drape so the opening's over your patient's perineal area. Again, take care not to contaminate your gloves.

7 Open the povidone-iodine solution package. Pour the solution on the cotton balls, as shown here.

8 Next, open up the lubricant packet. Squeeze the contents into one of the tray's compartments. Then, lubricate the first 3″ (7.6 cm) of the catheter.

9 If you're right-handed, separate Ms. Smith's labia with your *left* thumb and forefinger, as shown here. Keep your hand in this position until the catheter's inserted. Remember, this hand's now contaminated. Don't use it to touch anything sterile.

If your patient's obese, ask a coworker to hold the vaginal folds during the entire process.

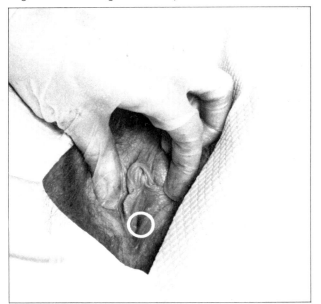

10 With your right hand, use the forceps to pick up a saturated cotton ball. Clean the right labia minora with a downward motion. Discard the used cotton ball into the wastebasket.

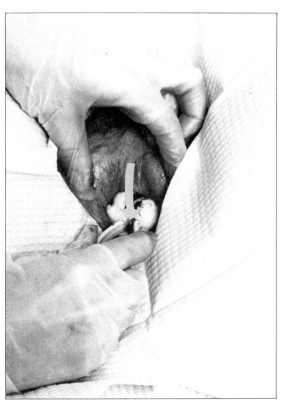

11 Using a clean cotton ball, repeat this procedure on the left labia minora.

Now, wipe between the labia minora over the urethral meatus, using another cotton ball. Take care not to confuse your patient's urethral meatus with her vaginal opening. If you can't see the urethral meatus, try exerting a slight downward pressure on her labia as you wipe with the cotton ball.

Continue cleaning the urethral meatus, using the remaining cotton balls.

12 Next, grasp the catheter with your right hand, as you would a dart. Gently insert the catheter 2″ to 3″ (5.1 to 7.6 cm) into Ms. Smith's urethral meatus.

Angle the catheter slightly upward as you advance it. Never force it. To make the insertion easier, ask your patient to exhale deeply while you advance the catheter.

Suppose the catheter won't pass into the bladder easily. Ask a coworker to obtain a smaller sterile catheter and try again. If you still have trouble inserting the catheter, notify the doctor.

Important: If you break aseptic technique for *any* reason, obtain a new pair of sterile gloves, or a new catheter tray (if necessary), and begin the procedure again.

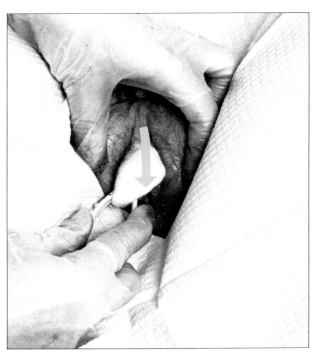

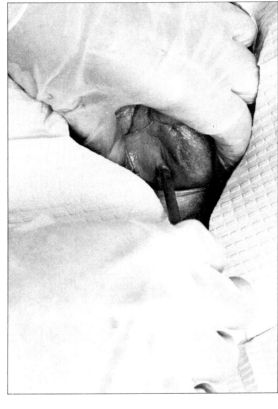

Culturing

Collecting a urine specimen using straight catheterization (for the female patient) continued

13 As the catheter enters your patient's bladder, urine will begin to drain. Place the free end of the catheter into the specimen container. Be sure to grasp the catheter end high enough to avoid contaminating the specimen.

Now, release the labia.

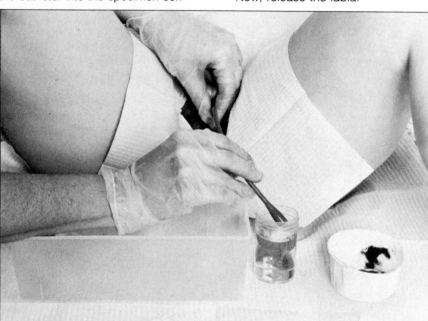

15 After all the urine's drained, remove the catheter. Dry your patient's perineum and help her into a comfortable position.

Place the lid on the specimen container. Then, remove your gloves and discard the entire catheter tray into a covered trash receptacle. Wash your hands.

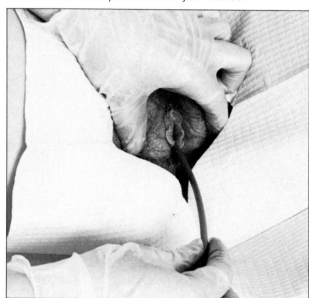

14 When the specimen container's three quarters full, drain the remaining urine into the kit's graduated container. Never allow more than 700 ml urine to drain or your patient may experience severe bladder spasms or go into shock.

What if your patient's bladder contains more than 700 ml of urine? Pinch off the catheter, remove it, and notify the doctor. He may want to recatheterize your patient at a later time.

Note: Some doctors may want all the urine drained. Check your hospital's policy.

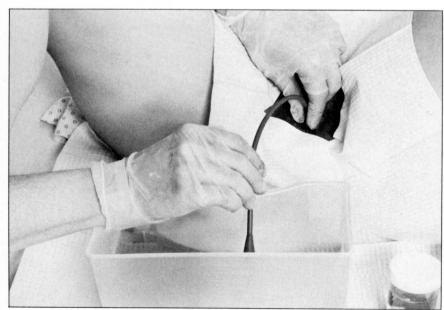

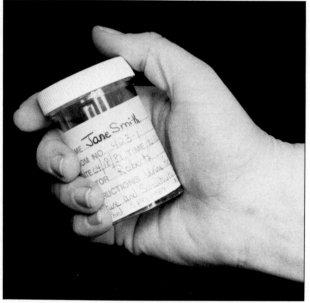

16 Label the urine specimen, noting the method of collection, and send it to the lab with the appropriate lab slip.

Then, document the procedure in your nurses' notes, including the amount of urine, its color and lucidity, as well as any sediment, odor, or blood clots. Also, record on your patient's intake and output record the amount of urine drained.

Collecting a urine specimen using straight catheterization (for the male patient)

1 *Suppose your male patient has a suspected urinary tract infection. The doctor may order a urine specimen collected by straight catheterization. (In some hospitals, the doctor performs this procedure.) Do you know how?*

First, ask your patient about any previous catheterizations. If he's had difficulty with them, notify the doctor. A urologist may have to perform the procedure.

Then, gather the following equipment: a sterile straight-catheter kit containing a straight catheter, a specimen container, lubricant, gloves, cotton balls, forceps, povidone-iodine (Betadine) solution, and drapes (see top photo). You'll also need: two bed-saver pads, washcloth, towel, soap, basin with warm water, and gloves (bottom photo).

If the doctor orders a different size catheter than the one supplied in the kit, be sure to obtain it before proceeding.

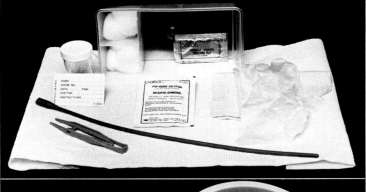

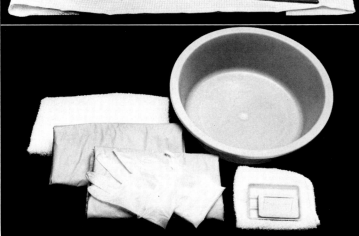

2 Wash your hands. Position the patient flat on his back. Place the bed-saver pad under his buttocks.

Suppose your patient can't lie on his back. Then, position him on his side.

Put on gloves before proceeding.

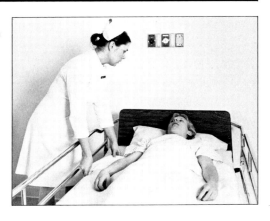

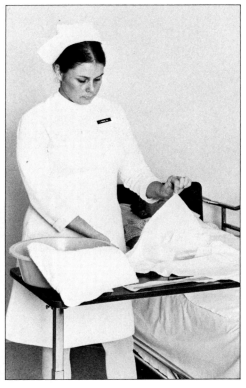

3 Next, using the washcloth, wash your patient's penis and perineal area with soap and water. Remember to use the same perineal cleaning procedure as the one described on pages 35 to 37. Pat the area dry.

Note: Retract your patient's foreskin if he's uncircumcised.

Replace the wet bed-saver pad with a dry one. Remove and discard your gloves.

Place the kit on the bedside table or overbed stand. Open the catheter kit, using aseptic technique, as the nurse is doing here. Then, put on the sterile gloves.

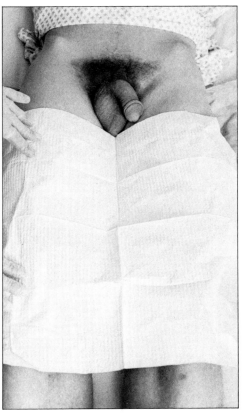

4 Place the sterile drape across your patient's thighs, as shown. Then, place the unopened precut sterile drape on top of it.

Culturing

Collecting a urine specimen using straight catheterization (for the male patient) continued

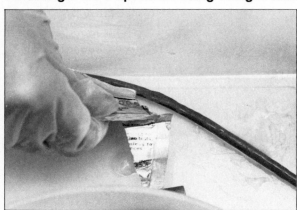

5 Now, open the packet of lubricant. Squeeze the contents into the tray compartment. (If the kit contains a syringe prefilled with lubricant, uncap the syringe.)
   Generously lubricate the first 7″ (17.8 cm) of the catheter. Keep the catheter in the lubricant until you're ready to insert it.

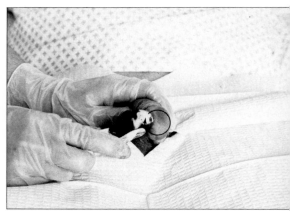

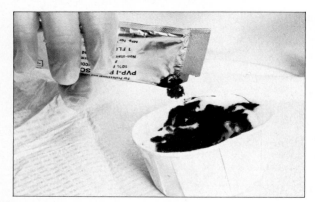

6 Next, open the povidone-iodine packet and pour the solution over the cotton balls.

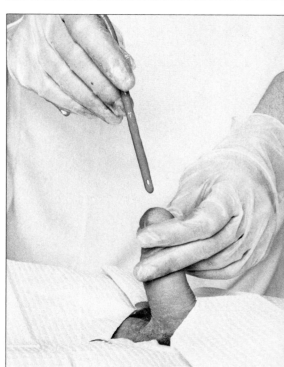

7 Open the precut drape. Then, position the drape over your patient's genital area. If you're right-handed, use your *left* hand to guide his penis through the drape's opening. Remember, this hand is now contaminated. Don't touch anything sterile with it.

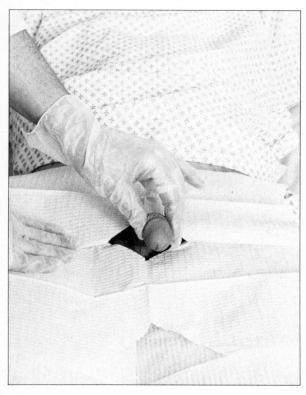

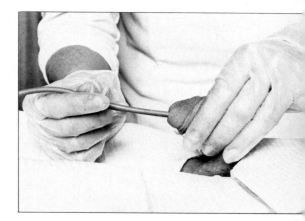

8 With your right hand, use the forceps to pick up a saturated cotton ball. Clean around the meatus in a circular motion. Wipe to the corona of the glans in a spiral motion. Discard the cotton ball.

Repeat this procedure, using all the cotton balls. Make sure no wisps of cotton remain on your patient's penis.

9 If your kit contains a syringe prefilled with lubricant, inject the lubricant into your patient's meatus. Then, remove the syringe and gently apply pressure around the meatus. This prevents lubricant from oozing out.

Then, use your left hand to hold your patient's penis at a 90° angle to his thighs. Grasp the catheter with your right hand, as you would a dart (see photo).

10 Insert the catheter into the meatus and advance it into the urethra. When you reach the prostate, you'll feel a slight resistance. Lower the penis to a 60° angle. Doing so changes the urethral curve, making passage around the prostate gland easier.

What if you can't pass the catheter around the prostate? Increase penis traction slightly and try again. If you're still unsuccessful, suspect an obstruction, remove the catheter, and notify the doctor.

Important: Never force a catheter. Doing so could perforate the patient's urethra.

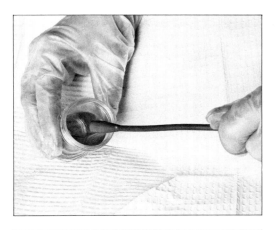

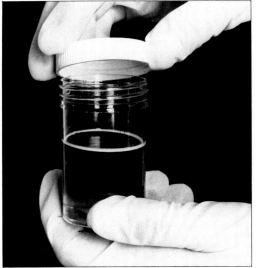

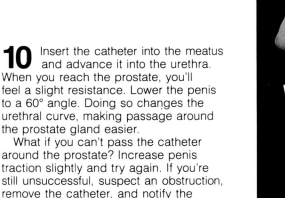

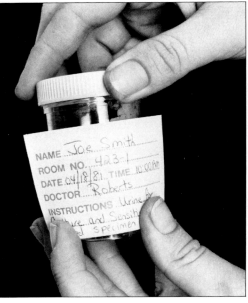

11 Now, place the open end of the catheter in the specimen cup. Urine will begin flowing when the catheter enters the bladder. Let the specimen cup fill three quarters full.

Drain the remaining urine into the kit's container. However, never drain more than 700 ml of urine or your patient may experience bladder spasms or go into shock.

If you suspect your patient still has more urine in his bladder, notify the doctor. He may want you to repeat the catheterization later to determine residual urine.

Note: Some doctors order all urine drained. Always follow hospital policy.

12 When the urine's drained, remove the catheter and dry your patient's perineum. Remember to pull your patient's foreskin forward if he's uncircumcised.

Cover the specimen container. Then, discard the catheter, and the entire catheter kit, in a covered trash receptacle.

13 Remove your gloves and discard them. Wash your hands. Label the specimen and send it to the lab with the appropriate lab slip. Then, document in your nurses' notes the quantity, color, and lucidity of the urine as well as any sediment, odor, or blood clots. Also, be sure to record on your patient's intake and output record the amount of urine obtained.

Culturing

Obtaining an endocervical canal culture

1 *Let's say 35-year-old Nancy Dubois arrives in the emergency department with signs of pelvic inflammatory disease (PID). The doctor wants you to take an endocervical canal culture. (However, in some hospitals, the doctor performs this procedure.) Here's how:*

Begin by gathering the following sterile equipment: vaginal speculum, culture swab with culture medium (we're using a Culturette), cotton balls, ring forceps, and gloves. You'll also need a gooseneck lamp.

Explain the procedure to Ms. Dubois. Tell her she may feel slight cramping when you insert the swab into her endocervical canal. But, assure her the cramping will be temporary.

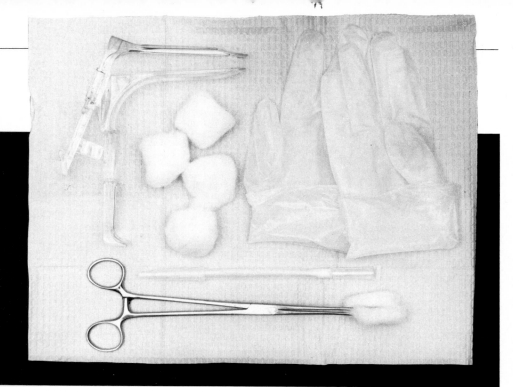

2 Now, place Ms. Dubois in the lithotomy position, as shown. Drape her thighs and symphysis pubis to protect her privacy. Make sure the lamp's positioned properly.

Wash your hands, and put on the gloves.

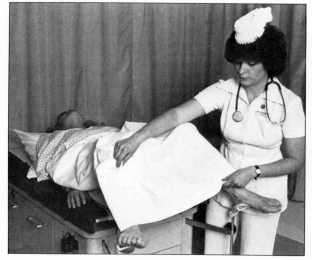

3 To make insertion easier, hold the speculum blades under running water. Don't apply a lubricant.

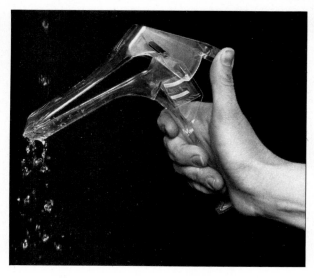

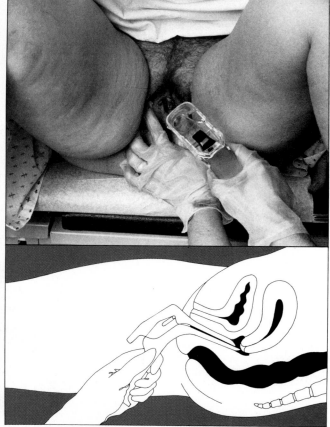

4 Then, spread apart your patient's labia. Carefully insert the speculum into her vagina (see top photo).

When you feel the speculum touch your patient's cervix, slowly open the blades by pressing the thumb lever (bottom illustration).

As you release your thumb, the lever will lock itself into position.

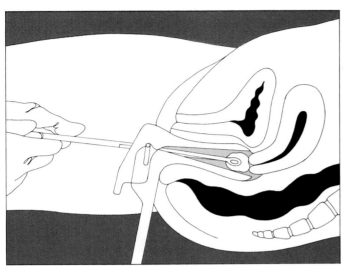

5 Now, using the sterile forceps, pick up a sterile cotton ball. Carefully insert the forceps into the vaginal canal and remove excess cervical mucus. Doing so will help you better see the cervical os. Then, discard the cotton ball into the wastebasket.

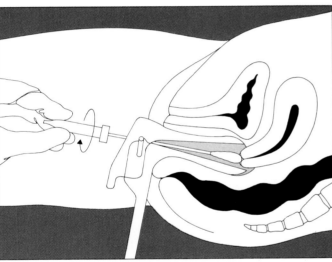

6 Remove the applicator swab from the culture medium tube. Then, insert the swab's cotton tip into your patient's endocervical canal. Gently rotate the swab from side to side for 10 to 30 seconds. This allows the swab to completely absorb any microorganisms present.

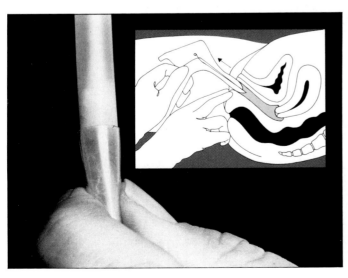

7 Now, withdraw the swab and place it in the culture medium tube.

Then, crush the ampule of culture medium at the base of the tube, as shown. Push the swab into the culture medium. Make sure it's completely immersed.

Remove the speculum (see inset). Help Ms. Dubois into a more comfortable position.

Label the specimen and send it to the lab immediately with the appropriate lab slip. Document the procedure.

Obtaining a stool specimen

Has the doctor ordered a stool culture for your patient? If so, you'll want to collect a specimen from your patient's first stool of the day. To do this, obtain a specimen container with glycerol-buffered saline solution in it. As you probably know, this solution prevents the stool from becoming acidic, which would affect the accuracy of laboratory analysis. *Salmonella* and *shigella* bacteria, for example, are undetectable in an acidified stool.

If your hospital doesn't have this type of specimen container, use a waterproof container with a tight-fitting lid, as provided by the lab. However, when using this type of container, be sure to send the stool specimen to the lab within 30 minutes after the patient defecates. If this isn't possible, place the specimen in the refrigerator. The specimen will become acidic if it's unrefrigerated.

To prepare for the procedure, tell your patient what you'll be doing and why. Answer any questions he may have. Then, ask him to urinate.

Place a clean bedside commode in his bathroom and instruct him to defecate into it.

Important: Never pour water or any other solution into the commode before or after the patient defecates. Doing so may affect specimen quality and lab results.

When he's done, use a tongue depressor to collect a walnut-sized stool specimen from the commode. Place the specimen in the container. Label the container with the appropriate slip and send it to the lab. Wash your hands thoroughly.

When taking a stool specimen for culture, follow these guidelines:
• If your patient has diarrhea, pour a small amount of the specimen directly into the container instead of using a tongue depressor.
• Have a nonambulatory patient urinate in a bedpan. Clean the bedpan and return it to your patient for a bowel movement.
• If your patient can't follow instructions, for example if he's an infant, insert a sterile swab past his anal sphincter. Rotate the swab several times and remove it. Place the swab into a sterile test tube.
• Place the specimen in a properly labeled container and send it to the lab as promptly as possible.

Culturing

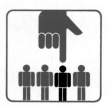

Collecting a stool specimen for ova and parasite testing

How do you obtain a stool specimen for ova and parasite testing? You'll take three separate stool specimens over a 7-day period. That way you will ensure specimen quality. Remember, parasites, if present, may not produce eggs daily. So, not every stool specimen will contain ova.

This photo shows the Para-Pak™ stool collection kit. Whichever kit you use, always follow the manufacturer's instructions.

Suppose the doctor needs test results more quickly? Collect a stool specimen on 3 consecutive days. But, be aware that the results may not be completely accurate.

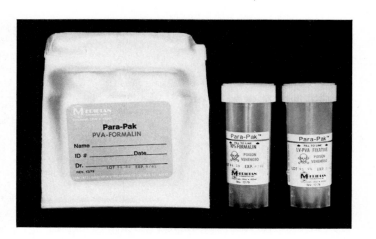

Obtaining an aerobic wound culture

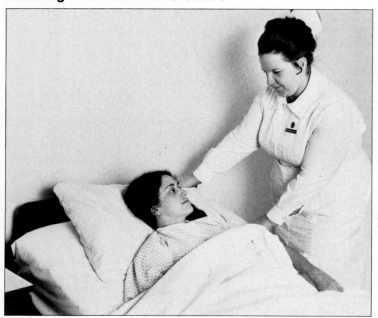

1 *Let's imagine 32-year-old Gina Felicetti has a two-week-old foot laceration that hasn't healed. After removing the dressing,* you discover signs of infection: inflammation, warmth, redness, and purulent discharge. After applying a clean, dry dressing, you notify the doctor. To determine the infection's cause, the doctor orders an aerobic culture of the wound. Do you know how to obtain this? If you're not sure, read this photostory.

Gather the following sterile equipment: culture swab with culture medium (we're using a Culturette® II), two packages of 4"x4" gauze pads, povidone-iodine (Betadine) swabs, normal saline solution or water, and a basin.

Now, explain the procedure to Ms. Felicetti. Remove the dressing to expose her wound.

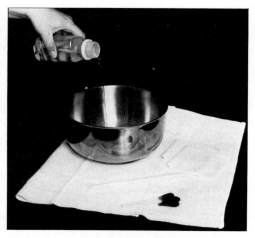

2 Wash your hands thoroughly. Using aseptic technique, remove the wrapper from the basin.

Then, open both 4"x4" gauze pad packages, the Culturette, and the povidone-iodine swabs, maintaining a sterile field.

Pour saline solution into the basin.

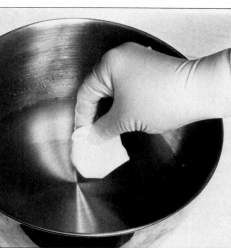

3 Put on the gloves. Dip a 4"x4" gauze pad into the saline solution. Then, carefully clean the wound, wiping from the wound's top to bottom. Discard the gauze pad. Using another saline-saturated pad, repeat this procedure until you've removed all of the gross debris.

Dry the wound with a dry sterile gauze pad.

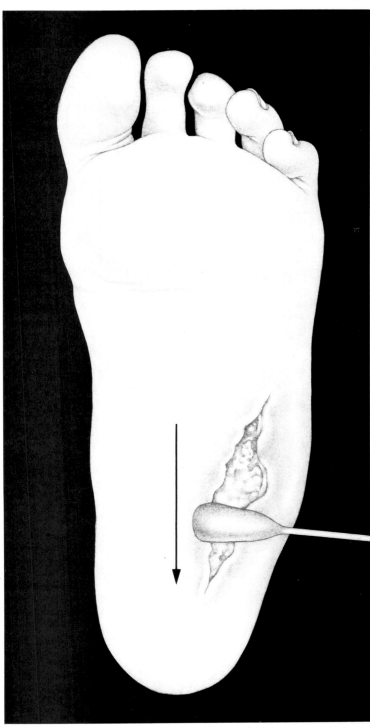

5 Remove the applicator swab from its container, being careful not to touch the sides (see inset).

Then, position the swab in the wound at the site of the most drainage. Collect as much of the drainage as possible.

Important: Don't collect a surface specimen, which affects the accuracy of the lab analysis.

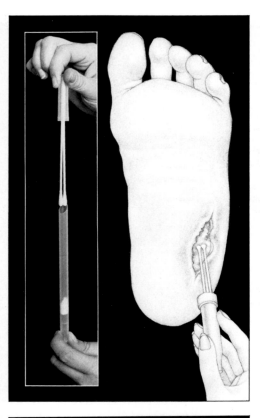
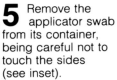

6 Now, return the swab to its container. Take care not to touch the outside of the container with the swab.

[Inset] Crush the culture-medium ampule at the base of the tube and push the swab into the medium. Make sure the swab's completely immersed.

Wash your hands. Then, properly label the specimen and appropriate lab slip. Remember to request a sensitivity test, if ordered. Send the specimen to the lab immediately. Never refrigerate the specimen.

Document the procedure in your nurses' notes.

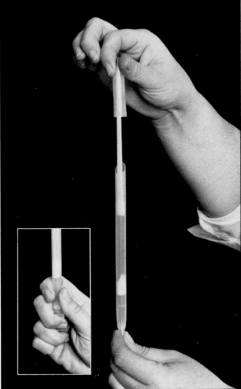

4 Next, wipe the wound with povidone-iodine swabs, again from the wound's top to bottom. Let the povidone-iodine solution dry. *Remember:* If your patient's allergic to iodine, alcohol swabs may be used to clean wounds for aerobic specimens. Warn the patient that alcohol will sting temporarily when applied directly to her open wound.

Culturing

Obtaining an anaerobic wound culture

1 *Suppose the doctor now wants an anaerobic culture from Ms. Felicetti's laceration. As you know, you can collect an anaerobic and an aerobic specimen for culture at either the same time or separately. (See pages 44 and 45 for aerobic culture guidelines.) Do you know how to collect an anaerobic specimen using an Anaerobic Culturette®? If you're unsure, read on:*

First, gather the necessary sterile equipment: 4"x4" gauze pads, normal saline solution, povidone-iodine (Betadine) swabs, basin, and gloves. You'll also need an Anaerobic Culturette, which contains a sterile rayon-tipped swab, sterile ampule with modified Cary-Blair transport medium, gas-generating tablet, ampule with activating solution, catalyst, two desiccants, polyester pledgets, and Bio-Bag™ with catalyst.

Then, explain to Ms. Felicetti what you're going to do and wash your hands.

Expose her foot laceration, and wash your hands again.

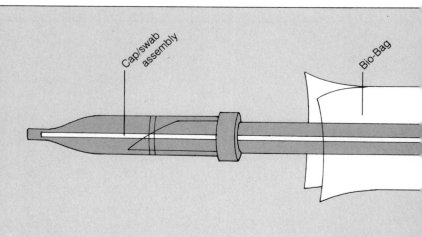

Cap/swab assembly

Bio-Bag

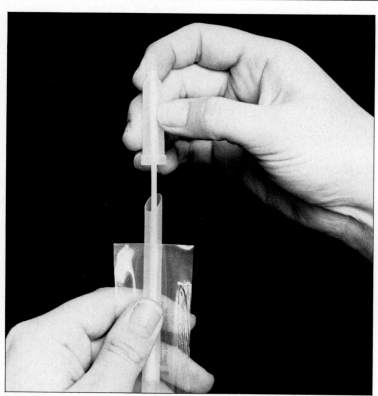

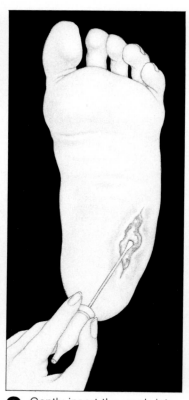

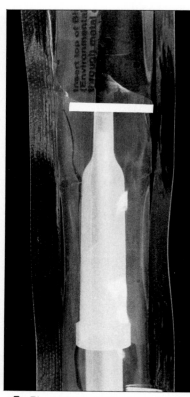

2 Now, open all your supplies using aseptic technique, and put on your sterile gloves. Clean the wound thoroughly, following the same procedure you used for the aerobic culture. Remove the sterile gloves.

Note: If you must separate the wound edges to obtain the specimen, keep your gloves on. Peel open the Culturette package, removing the Bio-Bag. Without removing the Culturette tube from the Bio-Bag, pull the Culturette cap (and attached swab) out of the bag, as the nurse is doing here. Be careful not to touch the side of the Bio-Bag with the cap or swab.

3 Gently insert the swab into the wound at the site that has the most drainage, and collect as much specimen as possible. Do not collect a surface specimen. Doing so will affect the accuracy of lab analysis.

4 Place the cap back on the Culturette tube. Then, applying gentle fingertip pressure to the cap, push the Culturette into the Bio-Bag until the top of the cap reaches the bag's line.

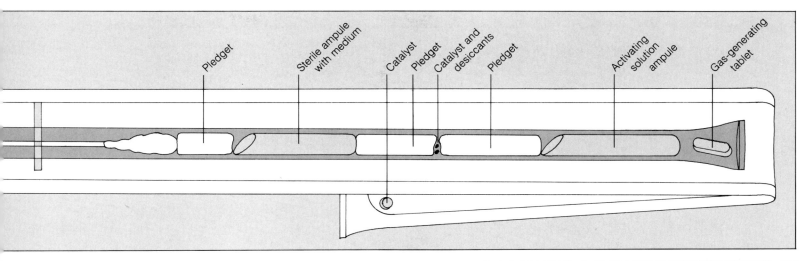

Pledget · Sterile ampule with medium · Catalyst · Pledget · Catalyst and desiccants · Pledget · Activating solution ampule · Gas-generating tablet

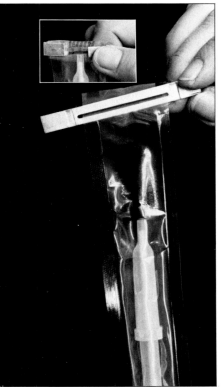

5 Now, pull the top of the Bio-Bag through the metal closure, as shown. (You'll find the closure under the bag's label.)

[Inset] Then, fold the top of the bag over the metal closure at least three times, until the closure reaches the line. Bend the closure ends so they are opposite the direction of the fold.

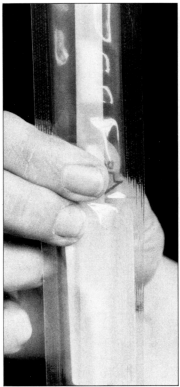

6 Invert the Bio-Bag so the Culturette cap is down. Then, with your fingers, crush the ampule closest to the swab. Doing so will allow transport medium to saturate the Culturette's pledget.

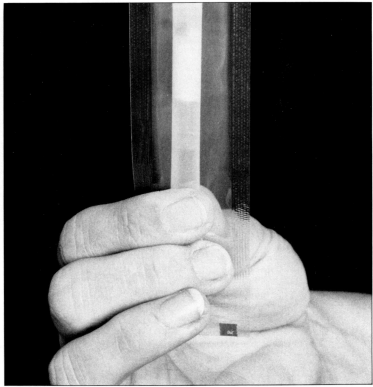

7 Invert the Bio-Bag so the Culturette cap is facing up. Crush the bottom ampule. Then, continue to hold the Bio-Bag upright until the tablet is completely dissolved. When the Bio-Bag inflates, you'll know you've done everything properly.

Important: Hydrogen gas is generated. Avoid exposure to spark or flame.

Label the Bio-Bag and the appropriate lab slip. Send the specimen to the lab immediately, and document the procedure in your nurses' notes.

Note: To remove the Culturette from the Bio-Bag, cut the bag at the line. Slide the Culturette up until the cap's exposed.

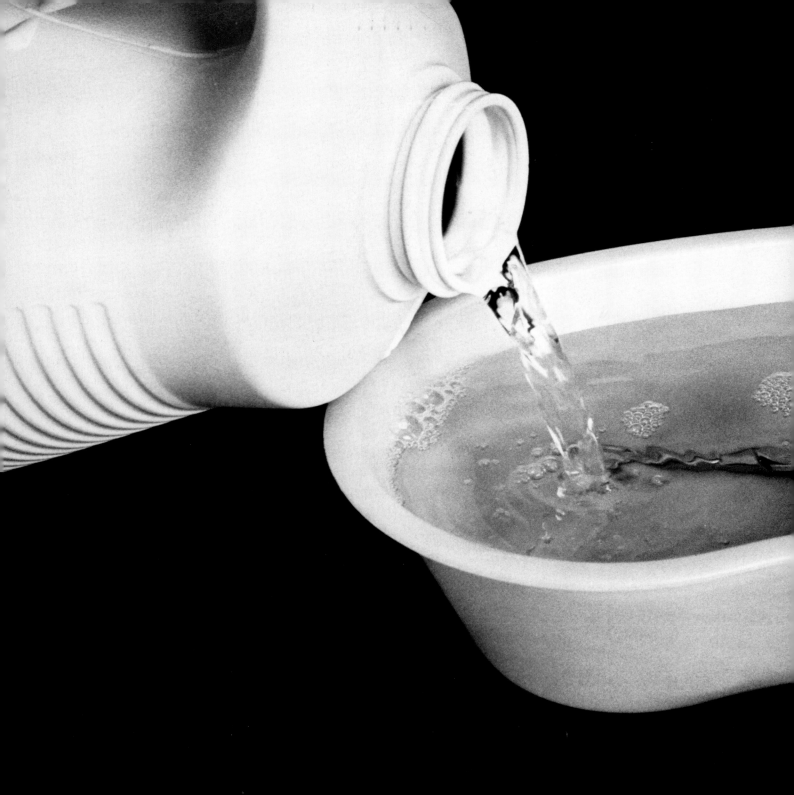

Preventing Infection

Immunization
Environmental considerations
Cleaning, disinfecting, and sterilizing

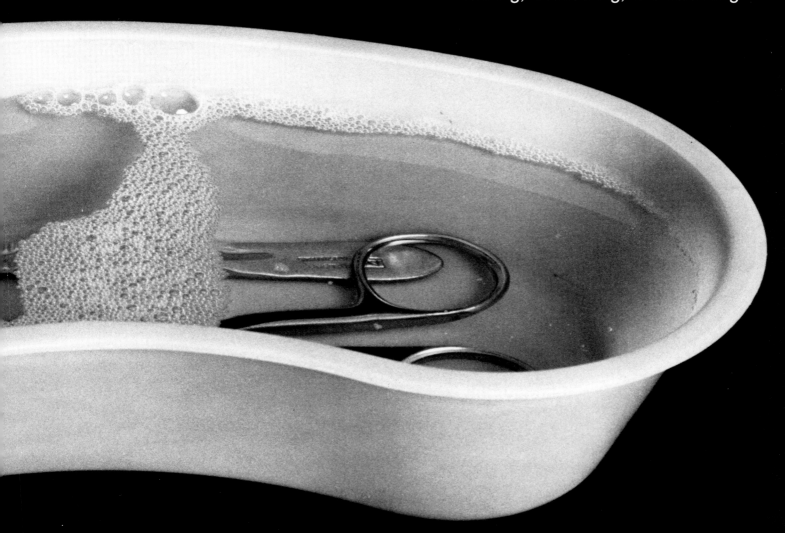

Immunization

To this point, we've reviewed fundamental microbiology and culturing techniques. On the following pages, we'll go one step further and take a look at immunization. Immunization, as you probably know, is one way to prevent infection.

When we discuss immunization, we're referring to the body's ability to form antibodies in response to an antigen. At one time or other, everyone comes in contact with at least one form of immunization.

How much do you need to know about immunization? On the pages that follow we'll tell you all you need to know before and after the procedure.

Identifying basic terms
Before you read further in this section on immunization procedures, review these common terms:

• *Antibody* - immune substance produced within the body in response to a specific antigen

---

• *Antigen* - substance capable of producing an immune response

---

• *Antitoxin* - immune serum that neutralizes or prevents action of toxin

---

• *Immunization* - vaccination or inoculation that protects a patient from a specific disease

---

• *Toxin* - a poisonous substance of animal or plant origin

• *Toxoid* - a specially treated toxin in which toxin properties are destroyed without affecting antibody-producing properties

Understanding immunity
When we discuss immunity, we're referring to the body's production of antibodies in response to antigens. This highly developed level of resistance is further categorized into two types: active and passive.

Active immunity is developed slowly (days or weeks) and lasts a long time (years, or even a lifetime). Active, like passive immunity, can be acquired by natural or artificial means. For example, a person who has had measles develops a resistance against recurrence of the disease. This resistance is known as *natural active immunity.* However, a person can develop a similar resistance without ever contracting measles. This resistance can be acquired by an injection of measles vaccine and is termed *artificial active immunity.*

Passive immunity, on the other hand, is quickly acquired and lasts a relatively short period of time (1 or 2 weeks). During fetal development, for example, globulin antibodies from the mother transfer to the fetus. So, a newborn's short-term disease resistance comes from *natural passive immunity.* Of course, the infant will receive only those immunities already acquired by the mother. Some of these immunities may be short lived.

Artificial passive immunity is established immediately by an immune serum injection, such as hepatitis B immune globulin human, or antirabies serum, equine.

Nurses' guide to routine immunizations

Is your patient scheduled for an immunization? If so, you'll want to know: which immunizations are considered routine, which physical conditions contraindicate immunization, and which complications may occur. On the next two pages, we've listed six routine immunizations. For guidelines on tuberculosis testing (often considered a routine immunization), see page 74. A more complete listing of immunizations appears in the NURSE'S GUIDE TO DRUGS™.

Note: Smallpox is no longer considered a routine immunization. The World Health Organization declared the world free of smallpox in May 1980.

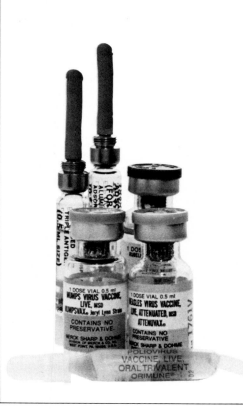

Rubella virus vaccine, live attenuated
Meruvax II*

Dosage
Adults, and children over 12 months: 0.5 ml (1,000 units) subcutaneously in outer aspect of upper arm. I.M. booster not recommended.

Side effects
Local: Pain, erythema, induration, lymphadenopathy
Other: Fever, rash, thrombocytopenic purpura, urticaria, arthritis, arthralgia, polyneuritis, anaphylaxis

Nursing considerations
• Contraindicated during immunosuppressive drug therapy; immunodeficiency conditions; active, untreated tuberculosis; fever; pregnancy. Use cautiously if patient has hypersensitivity to neomycin sulfate (Myciguent), chickens, ducks, eggs, or feathers. Defer in acute illness.
• Obtain accurate history of allergies, especially to ducks, rabbits, and antibiotics, as well as past reaction to immunization.
• Never give within 3 months of administration of immune serum globulin, blood, or plasma: antibodies in serum may interfere with immune response.
• Warn patient to avoid getting pregnant during first 3 months after immunization.
• Have epinephrine 1:1,000 available in case of anaphylaxis.
• Vaccine may temporarily suppress tuberculin skin-test reaction.
• Avoid administering other live virus vaccines for at least 1 month, if possible.
• Store vaccine in refrigerator and protect it from light. Solution may be used if red, pink, or yellow; however, discard if it becomes cloudy.
• Use only diluent supplied. Discard vaccine 8 hours after reconstituting it.

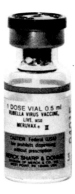

Poliovirus (Sabin) vaccine, live, oral, trivalent
Orimune

Dosage
Children over 6 weeks: Routine primary polio vaccination for adults is unnecessary except when the risk of exposure to poliovirus is increased, such as travel to areas where poliovirus is epidemic or endemic; employment in laboratory with poliovirus; employment in close contact with patients possibly excreting poliovirus; and residence in areas where wild poliovirus is reported. Recommended dosage is 0.5 ml in prepackaged vial. Repeat dose in 8 weeks. Administer third dose 12 months after second dose.
Booster: Contents of plastic vial; 2 drops or 0.5 ml orally

Side effects
In rare cases, paralysis of recipient or contacts

Nursing considerations
• Contraindicated during immunosuppressive drug therapy, immunodeficiency conditions.
• Obtain accurate history of allergies, as well as past reactions to immunizations.
• Defer in acute illness, fever, vomiting, or diarrhea.
• Never give within 3 months of immune serum globulin, blood, or plasma administration: antibodies in serum may interfere with immune response.
• Keep vaccine frozen until used. You may refrigerate thawed, unopened vial for up to 30 days. Opened vials may be refrigerated up to 7 days.
• Solution may be used if it turns red, pink, or yellow.
• Avoid administering other live virus vaccines (except measles, or diphtheria, pertussis, and tetanus) for at least 1 month, if possible.
• Recommend vaccine recipient avoid household contact with immunodeficient people for 2 to 3 weeks.
• While the activated oral trivalent (Sabin) poliovirus vaccine is usually the preferred vaccine for children, the inactivated (Salk) poliovirus vaccine is recommended for adult immunization. In adults, the risk of vaccine-associated paralysis is lower in the Salk vaccine. Follow manufacturer's instructions when administering vaccine.

Measles (rubeola) virus vaccine, live attenuated
Attenuvax*

Dosage
Adults and children 15 months or older: 0.5 ml (1,000 units) subcutaneously on outer aspect of upper arm. Booster not recommended.

Side effects
Local: Erythema, swelling, tenderness
Other (within 5 to 10 days): Fever and rash, lymphadenopathy, anaphylaxis, anorexia, leukopenia, febrile convulsions in susceptible children

Nursing considerations
• Contraindicated during immunosuppressive drug therapy, immunodeficiency conditions, pregnancy, fever. Use cautiously if patient has hypersensitivity to neomycin sulfate (Myciguent), chickens, ducks, eggs, or feathers.
• Obtain accurate history of allergies (especially to eggs), as well as past reactions to immunizations. Defer in acute illness.
• Never give within 3 months of immune serum globulin, blood, or plasma administration: antibodies in serum may interfere with immune response.
• Warn patient to avoid getting pregnant during first 3 months after immunization.
• Keep epinephrine 1:1,000 available in case of anaphylaxis.
• Store vaccine in refrigerator and protect it from light. Solution may be used if red, pink, or yellow; however, discard if it becomes cloudy.
• Use only diluent supplied. Discard vaccine 8 hours after reconstituting it.
• Vaccine may temporarily suppress tuberculin skin-test reaction.
• Avoid administering other live virus vaccine (except for oral polio and mumps vaccines), for at least 1 month.

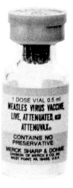

*Available in both the United States and in Canada

Immunization

Nurses' guide to routine immunizations continued

Diphtheria and tetanus toxoids and pertussis vaccine (DPT) adsorbed
Tri-Immunol

Dosage
Children ages 6 weeks to 6 years: 0.5 ml
I.M. on midlateral thigh or deltoid muscles.
Administer vaccine doses 2 months apart
for three doses and a fourth dose 1 year
later. Avoid injecting same muscle site more
than once.
Booster: 0.5 ml I.M. before school entry.
Effective for 10 years

Side effects
Local: Sore, red nodule remaining several
weeks
Other: Slight fever, chills, malaise, encephalopathy, anaphylaxis

Nursing considerations
• Contraindicated during immunosuppressive drug therapy, fever, convulsions,
neurologic disorders. Defer in acute illness.
• Obtain accurate history of allergies, as
well as past reactions to immunizations.
• Keep epinephrine 1:1,000 available
in case of anaphylaxis.
• Not to be used for active infection.
• Shake vial well before using. Store in
refrigerator, according to manufacturer's
instructions.

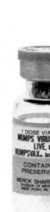

Mumps vaccine, live attenuated
Mumpsvax*

Dosage
*Mumps-susceptible adults, and children age
1 to puberty:* 1 vial (1,000 units) subcutaneously in outer aspect of upper arm. Booster
not recommended.

Side effects
Local: Erythema
Other: Urticaria, anaphylaxis, fever, rash,
regional lymphadenopathy

Nursing considerations
• Contraindicated during immunosuppressive drug therapy, immunodeficiency
conditions, pregnancy, fever. Use cautiously
if patient has hypersensitivity to neomycin
sulfate (Myciguent), chickens, eggs, or
feathers.
• Obtain accurate history of allergies (especially to chickens, feathers, and antibiotics), as well as past reactions to immunizations. Defer in active infection.
• Never give within 3 months of immune
serum globulin, blood, or plasma administration: antibodies in serum may interfere
with immune response.
• Keep epinephrine 1:1,000 available in
case of anaphylaxis.
• Store vaccine in refrigerator and protect it
from light. Solution may be used if red,
pink, or yellow; however, discard if it becomes cloudy.
• Use only diluent supplied. Discard vaccine
8 hours after reconstituting it.
• Avoid administering other live virus vaccines (except measles) for at least 1 month,
if possible.
• Vaccine may temporarily suppress tuberculin skin-test reaction.

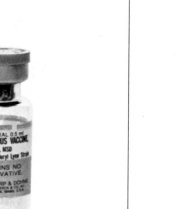

Diphtheria and tetanus toxoids, combined

Dosage
Adults and children ages 6 and up: 0.5 ml
I.M. 4 to 6 weeks apart for two doses and a
third dose 1 year later.
Booster: 0.5 ml I.M. every 10 years.
Children under age 6: **Pediatric plain toxoid:**
0.5 ml subcutaneously 4 to 6 weeks apart
for three doses; fourth dose 1 year later.
Pediatric absorbed toxoid: 0.5 ml I.M. 4 to
8 weeks apart for two doses and a third
dose 6 to 12 months later
Booster: 0.5 ml before school entry

Side effects
Local: Stinging, edema, erythema, pain,
induration
Other: Chills, fever, malaise, anaphylaxis

Nursing considerations
• Contraindicated during immunosuppressive drug therapy, immunodeficiency
conditions, or fever. Defer in any acute
illness, except in emergency.
• Use single antigen during polio risks. For
children under age 6, use only when
diphtheria, tetanus, and pertussis combination is contraindicated because of pertussis
component.
• Be sure toxoid is the appropriate strength.
• Obtain accurate history of allergies, as
well as past reactions to immunizations.
• Keep epinephrine 1:1,000 available
in case of anaphylaxis.
• Don't use hot or cold compresses on the
injection site: they may increase severity
of local reaction.

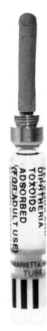

Giving immunizations

Are you administering an immunization to your patient? If so, follow these guidelines carefully and observe your patient closely:
- Check the doctor's order.
- Obtain an accurate patient history. Be sure it includes information about any present febrile illness; allergic reaction to antibiotics or past immunizations; immune deficiency condition of patient or other household members; and past childhood diseases, such as mumps or measles.
- Explain to the patient how and why the vaccine is administered, and provide information about possible side effects.
- Obtain a signed consent form.
- Check the vaccine label for dosage, route, and preparation instructions. Also, note the expiration date. If the vaccine is outdated, return it to the pharmacy, and obtain new vaccine.
- Check the vaccine's color and consistency. If you have any questions, check with the pharmacist before administering it.
- Prepare the vaccine (and store the unused portion), following manufacturer's instructions.
- Recheck vaccine label for dosage, route, and preparation instructions.
- Check patient's arm band to reconfirm identity.
- Administer vaccine, following manufacturer's instructions.
- Document vaccine administration, including type, manufacturer and lot number, route, dosage, site, date, and time.
- Give patient or responsible family member an immunization record.

Administering a subcutaneous injection

1 *Are you administering a vaccine subcutaneously? If so, follow these steps:*
Begin by gathering the following equipment: the ordered vaccine (Pneumovax*), several alcohol wipes; a 1 cc, 25G tuberculin syringe with a ⅝" needle attached; and an assortment of other needles (25G to 27G and ½" to 1" in length, not shown).

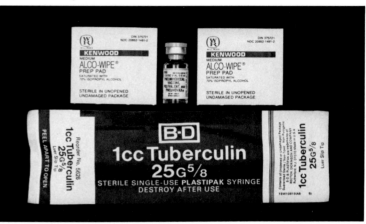

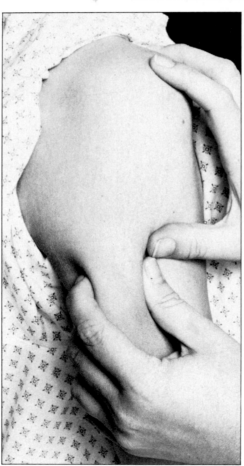

2 Next, select an injection site. In this photo, the nurse has selected the upper outer aspect of her arm. To locate the site exactly, position the patient's arm by her side, inner aspect up. Then, measure about 4" (10.2 cm) down from the top of her shoulder and a third of the way around her arm.

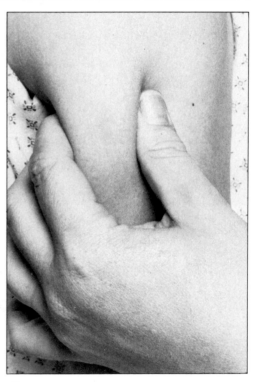

3 To determine the proper needle size, use your thumb and forefinger to gently pinch a fold of skin at the injection site. Carefully measure the distance from the fold's base to its crest. If the fold measures more or less than ⅝" (1.6 cm), remove the ⅝" needle that's on the syringe and replace it with one that's closer to the correct length. (You'll probably need a ½" needle for a child or a thin patient, and a ⅞" or 1" needle for an obese patient.)
By using a needle that's the correct length, you ensure injecting the vaccine into subcutaneous tissue. You also spare your patient unnecessary pain.

Immunization

Administering a subcutaneous injection continued

4 Now, examine the vaccine vial, its label, and contents. Be sure the solution's the proper color and consistency, and not outdated. Remove the protective cap from the vial, as shown here.

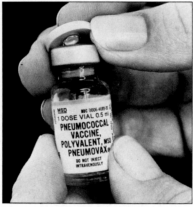

5 Clean the top of the vial with an alcohol swab, as the nurse is doing here.

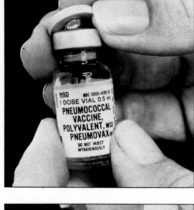

6 Draw up 0.5 ml into the syringe, as the nurse is doing here. Cap the syringe.

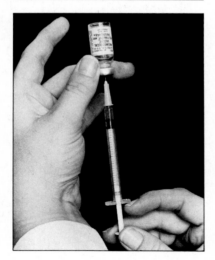

7 Using a circular motion, clean the injection site thoroughly with an alcohol swab. Allow the skin to dry completely before you proceed, to ensure that all microorganisms are killed. Remember, if you inject the vaccine when the skin's still wet, you may introduce some of the alcohol into the subcutaneous tissue.

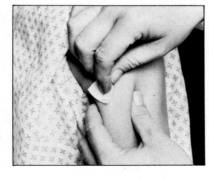

8 Firmly grasp the skin, as the nurse is doing in this photo. Then, position the needle bevel up. If you're injecting with a ½" needle, hold it at a 90° angle to the skin. If you're using a ⅝" or longer needle, position it at a 45° angle, as shown here.

Quickly insert the needle. Once it's inserted, release your grasp on the patient's skin. If you don't, you'll inject vaccine into the compressed skin and tissue, which will irritate nerve fibers, causing discomfort.

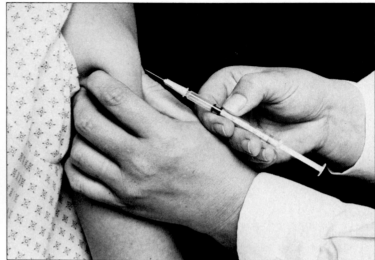

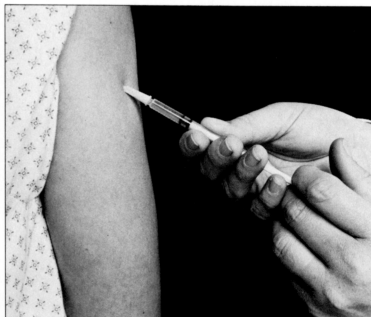

9 Now, check needle placement by pulling back on the syringe plunger. If blood enters the syringe, quickly withdraw the needle and place an alcohol swab over the site. Discard everything and begin again.

Suppose no blood enters the syringe. Then, begin injecting the vaccine slowly. Never inject rapidly; doing so puts unnecessary pressure on the tissue and causes pain.

10 When you're finished injecting the vaccine into your patient's arm, place an alcohol swab over the site. Carefully withdraw the needle at the same angle you inserted it. As you do, use the swab to apply pressure to the site. This will help seal punctured tissue and prevent the vaccine from seeping out.

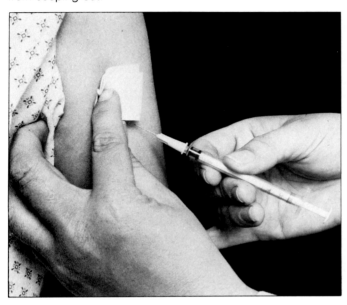

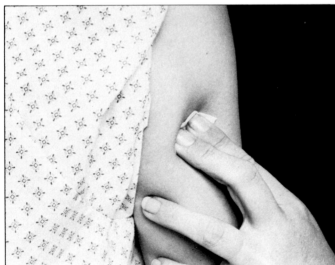

11 Now, massage the injection site with a clean alcohol swab. This helps distribute the vaccine, promoting quick absorption.

Immediately observe your patient for adverse side effects and observe her for up to 30 minutes afterward.

Finally, document in your notes the procedure and your patient's reaction to it. Be sure to include the type of vaccine, manufacturer and lot number, dosage, route, site, time and date administered, and your initials. Give your patient a record of the vaccination. Then, dispose of all equipment according to your hospital's policy.

Administering an I.M. injection with a Tubex® syringe

1 *Are you administering a tetanus toxoid injection with a Tubex® syringe? If you are, you'll need a Tubex holder, a prefilled glass syringe with an attached needle and rubber protector, and several alcohol swabs.*

Depending on the vaccine you'll be using and your patient's age, the glass syringe will come filled with the proper dosage. After rechecking the dosage, the expiration date, the syringe, and your patient's name and age, follow these steps:

First, explain the procedure to your patient and reassure her. Then, wash your hands. Remember to maintain aseptic technique throughout this procedure.

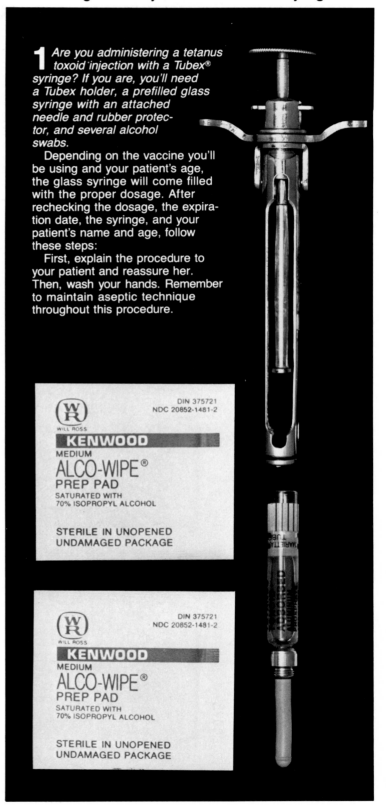

Immunization

Administering an I.M. injection with a Tubex® syringe continued

2 Next, unlock the Tubex plunger. Firmly, pull the plunger up as far as it will go (see photo).

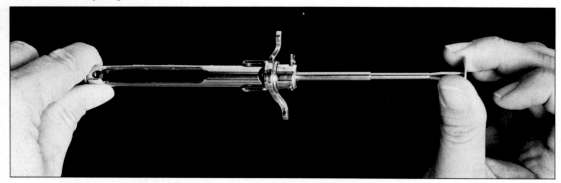

3 Holding the plunger with one hand, flip the top of the Tubex holder to one side, as the nurse is doing here.

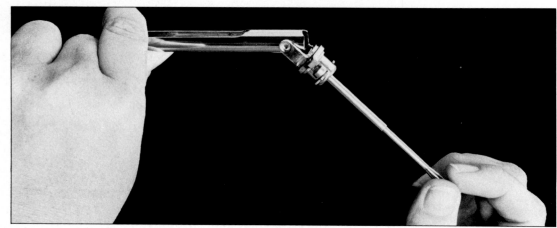

4 Now, insert the prefilled glass syringe—needle down—into the Tubex holder.
Flip up the plunger top. Then, lock the Tubex plunger in place.

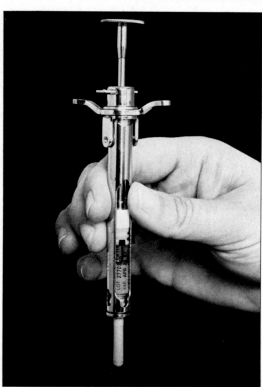

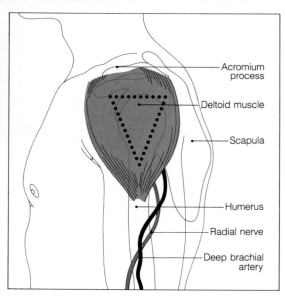

Acromium process

Deltoid muscle

Scapula

Humerus

Radial nerve

Deep brachial artery

5 If you decide to use the deltoid muscle area of your patient's arm for the injection, you can locate the area by studying the shaded triangle in this illustration.
Caution: Take care to stay within these boundaries. If you inject outside this area, you risk damaging the radial nerve.

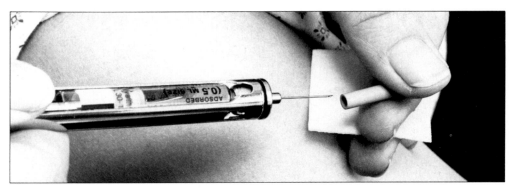

6 Next, using an alcohol wipe, clean an area 2″ (5.1 cm) in diameter around the injection site, moving from the center outward in a circular motion. This swabbing kills any microorganisms present on the skin. Be sure to let the alcohol dry completely before you proceed.

Then, place the alcohol swab between two of your fingers for later use, as shown here. Remove the rubber protector from the needle.

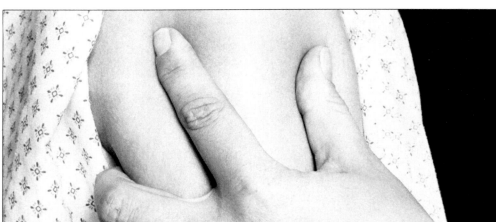

7 With one hand, firmly stretch the skin around the injection site until it's taut. Doing so makes needle insertion easier and displaces subcutaneous tissue, and helps disperse the vaccine solution quicker.

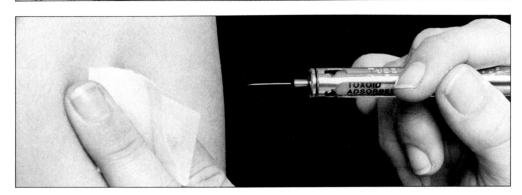

8 Now, use your other hand to hold the syringe, as the nurse is doing here. Keep the syringe horizontal until you're ready to inject the vaccine.

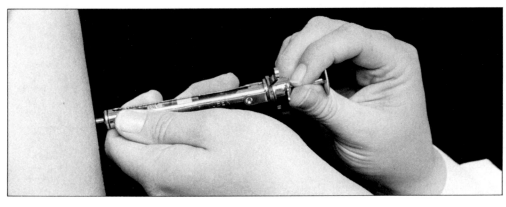

9 Insert the needle at a 90° angle to the skin, using a quick, dartlike motion. As you enter the muscle, expect to feel some resistance.

To confirm needle placement, gently pull back on the Tubex plunger. If there's blood in the glass syringe, you may have entered a vein. Withdraw the needle. Remove and discard the needle and the prefilled glass syringe (see page 58). Replace the prefilled glass syringe and needle with new ones, and try again.

But, if no blood appears, the needle's placed properly.

Immunization

Administering an I.M. injection with a Tubex® syringe continued

10 Holding the needle steady, inject the vaccine at a slow, even rate. Quick, unsteady movements will hurt your patient, traumatize tissue, and cause improper vaccine distribution.

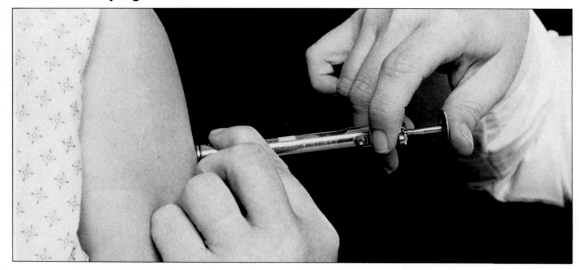

11 When you finish injecting the vaccine, withdraw the needle rapidly. Then, use the alcohol swab to apply pressure to the injection site. Watch your patient closely for adverse reactions.

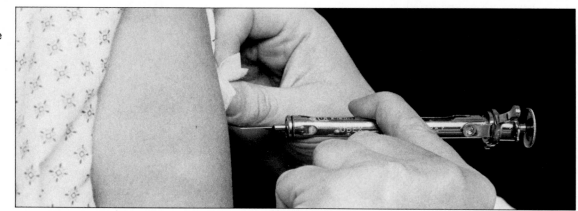

12 Now, cut off the needle, as shown in this photo. Discard the needle in the proper receptacle.

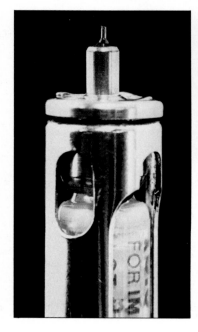

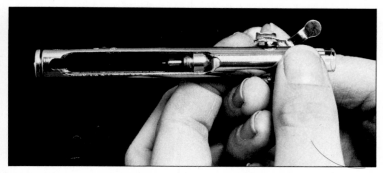

13 To remove the empty glass syringe from the Tubex holder, unlock the plunger. Then, pull the plunger up as far as it will go and flip the top to one side. Remove the glass syringe. Then, dispose of the glass syringe, according to your hospital's policy.

Warn your patient that the injection site may become hard and warm. Also tell her that her arm may feel stiff, but that she should exercise her arm as she would normally.

Finally, document the following information in your notes: time, date, vaccine administered, manufacturer and lot number, route, site, amount, patient's reaction, and your initials. Give your patient a record of the vaccination.

Patient teaching

Home care

Immunizing your child

Dear Parent:
Consider immunizing your child an effective form of health insurance. Here is a recommended schedule for protecting your child against polio, measles, mumps, rubella, diphtheria, pertussis (whooping cough), and tetanus. *Note:* While the tuberculin test is actually a diagnostic skin test, the results should be part of your child's record.

Letting your child miss one or more of these immunizations means needless risk of serious illness, perhaps with life-threatening complications.

Vaccination time-line

Age	Immunization
2 months	First dose: diphtheria/tetanus/pertussis vaccine; polio vaccine
4 months	Second dose: diphtheria/tetanus/pertussis vaccine; polio vaccine
6 months	Third dose: diphtheria/tetanus/pertussis vaccine
15 months	Single dose: rubella vaccine; measles vaccine; mumps vaccine; tuberculin test
18 months	Fourth dose: diphtheria/tetanus/pertussis vaccine; third dose: polio vaccine
4-5 years	Fifth dose: diphtheria/tetanus/pertussis vaccine; fourth dose: polio vaccine

For your easy reference, we've provided a documentation record below. As you know, the effectiveness of any immunization program depends on your cooperation. Be sure your child receives each immunization on schedule. In addition, keep accurate records of each immunization date, noting your child's reaction.

Child's name: _____

Immunization checklist for your child's protection

Type	Dose	Date	Reaction
Polio	1st		
	2nd		
	3rd		
	4th		
DPT	1st		
	2nd		
	3rd		
	4th		
	5th		
Measles	One time only		
Mumps	One time only		
Rubella	One time only		
Tuberculin test	Type		

Environmental considerations

You may not realize it, but you're already familiar with many environmental considerations that control or prevent infection. Every time you make a bed, dispose of soiled linen, or fill a water carafe properly, you're controlling possible infection. Over the following pages, you'll learn about other environmental considerations, including employee health and patient education.

Want to find out more? Read the next few pages.

Understanding linen storage procedures

Of course, linen storage procedures vary from hospital to hospital. But let's assume that linen storage is the responsibility of the laundry department personnel in your hospital. Every day a laundry aide comes to your unit to deliver and store a properly covered supply of linen that's been washed, dried, ironed, and folded.

Sound basic? Sure, but it's worth consideration, because this process is one way infection can be prevented. Improper linen storage or distribution can spread contaminants throughout the hospital. As a result, patients may needlessly develop infections.

So, you must understand how your linen system works. The steps listed here will reacquaint you with the proper linen storage and distribution procedures.

Reviewing infection basics: Making a bed

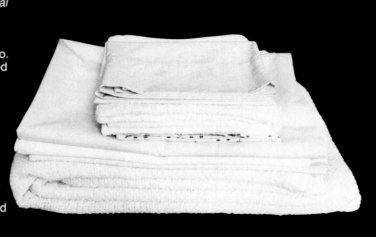

1 *Making a bed. You probably do it several times a day, and several hundred times a month. But did you know that something as simple as making a bed can be part of infection control? Read the following photostory to find out how.*

Picture this: The patient in room 310 was discharged 2 hours ago. At that time you stripped the bed, disposed of the linen, and removed the bedpan and other articles from the bedside cabinet. After that, a housekeeping staff member scrubbed the bed's waterproof, insectproof mattress cover with a disinfecting agent and water (following hospital policy).

When the mattress cover dries, here's how to proceed:

First, obtain the bed linen and towels you'll need from the linen storage area. Depending on your hospital, these linens may be called a discharge pack. In most cases, the pack includes: a bedspread, a top sheet, bottom sheet, pillowcase, towel, washcloth, and patient gown.

Set the discharge pack on a clean, dry area, such as the overbed table.

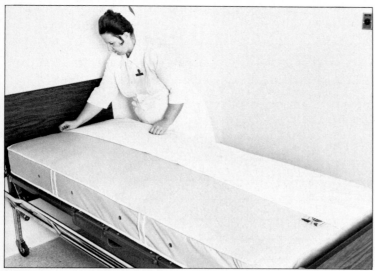

2 Now, standing at the side of the bed, place the bottom sheet over one half of the mattress cover, as the nurse is doing here. To help reduce dust-particle activity, make only half of the bed at a time, and *never* shake the sheets over the bed.

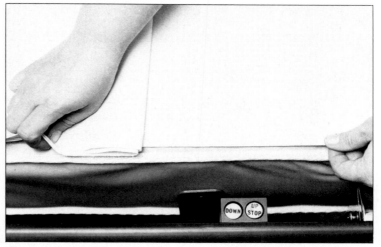

3 Position the sheet's bottom edge even with the foot of the mattress.

Carefully unfold the bottom sheet, keeping the hemmed edge against the mattress, away from the patient. The sheet's top edge will hang 8″ to 10″ (20.3 to 25 cm) over the head of the mattress. Tuck in the sheet at the top.

- Depending on the number of beds in your unit, a daily supply of linen is loaded onto a cart by a laundry aide.
- The aide covers the cart with a color-coded, moisture-resistant nylon drape. The drape also has a front flap.
- The drape keeps the linen free of airborne contaminants and moisture.
- The color coding helps the aide determine the cart's destination. For example, linen that's bound for the ICU may be color coded with a blue drape.

At this point, the laundry aide wheels the cart into the clean utility room or storage area of your unit.

Do you need linen? If so, lift up the drape's front flap. Remove only the linens needed at this time. Immediately replace the drape. Remember, never store or hoard linen on your unit or in your patient's room.

But where does the job of laundry personnel end and your job begin? Your responsibility is to make sure a clean linen supply arrives on your unit daily; a two-day linen supply arrives on Saturday or the day before a holiday; the linen is properly covered; and that the day's leftover linen is returned to the laundry for inventory.

As you know, additional linen, if needed, may be obtained by submitting a requisition slip to the laundry department. On Sundays and holidays you may need to send a requisition slip to the central supply department.

---

4 Miter the sheet's top corner, as shown. Tuck the sheet's mitered corner under the mattress as far as possible.

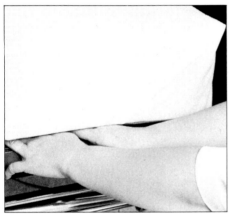

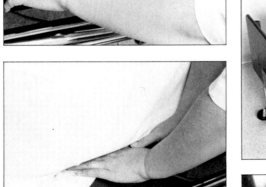

5 Then, tightly tuck the entire side of the sheet under the mattress, moving from the top mattress corner to the bottom mattress corner.

Note: Does your hospital use fitted bottom sheets? Fit the top left sheet corner over the top left mattress corner.

Tightly tuck the entire side of the sheet under the mattress, moving from the top left corner to the bottom left corner. Fit the bottom left sheet corner over the bottom left mattress corner.

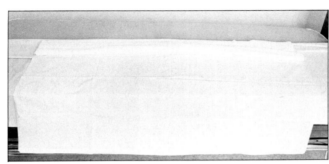

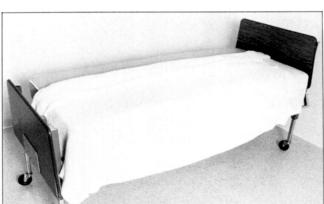

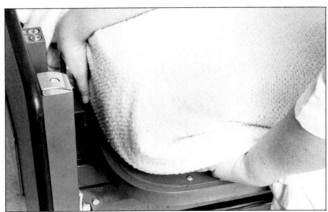

6 If you're using a drawsheet, position it over the bottom sheet, midway between the head and foot of the bed.

Unfold the drawsheet toward you. Tightly tuck the drawsheet's side under the mattress.

7 Next, lay the top sheet over the drawsheet. Then, unfold the top sheet, hemmed edge up, making sure 8″ to 10″ (20.3 to 25 cm) hangs over the foot of the mattress.

Next, place the top of spread 5″ to 8″ (12.7 to 20.3 cm) below the edge of the sheet.

Later, you'll pull the top edge of the spread and sheet over the pillow.

Note: In some hospitals, you'll fold down about 14″ (36 cm) of the spread. Later, you'll place the pillow in this space, and pull the spread over the pillow.

8 Tuck the top sheet and spread under the foot of the mattress, as the nurse is doing in this photo.

Environmental considerations

Reviewing infection basics: Making a bed continued

9 Miter the bottom corner of the top sheet and spread, as shown here.
  Repeat the entire procedure on the other side of the bed.

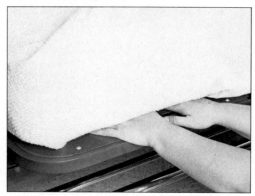

12 Now, as you fit pillow into pillowcase, firmly push the corners of the pillow into the corners of the pillowcase. Be careful not to let the pillow or pillowcase touch your uniform. Never hold the pillow under your chin.

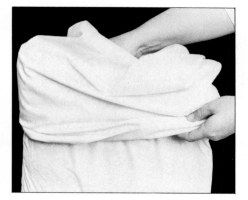

10 Now you're ready to put the pillow in the pillowcase. To do this, first unfold the pillowcase. Then, use one hand to hold the pillowcase by the bottom seam. Use your other hand to gather the entire length of the pillowcase, as shown here.

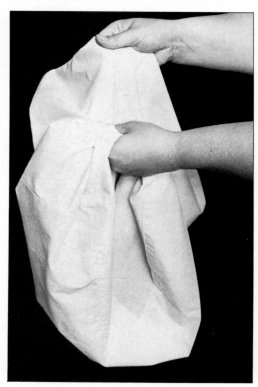

13 If necessary, make an envelope fold in the pillowcase's side seam so the case fits tightly.

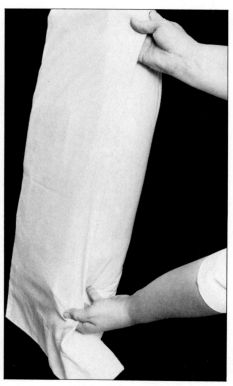

11 With one hand, grasp the gathered pillowcase by the bottom seam, and hold the pillow so the zipper is facing toward you.

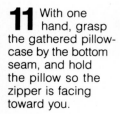

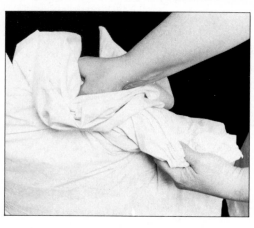

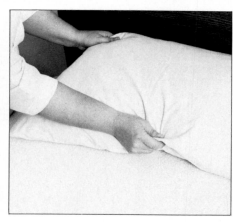

14 Place the pillow on the bed. Make sure the open end of the pillowcase is away from the door.
  Finally, hang the towel and washcloth inside the bedside cabinet, or in your patient's bathroom, according to hospital policy. Remember, always wash your hands before beginning patient care.

How to care for soiled linen

1 *As a nurse, you're well acquainted with the procedure for changing soiled linens. But, did you know that by performing the procedure properly you can help prevent the spread of infection? Use this photostory as a guide:*

Note: The nurse in these photos will be using a color-coded (by nursing unit) hamper bag, and metal stand with a foot-operated lid. If this equipment is unavailable, follow your hospital's linen removal policy using other equipment.

To prevent cross-contamination, first wash your hands with soap and warm, running water. Open the hamper stand by stepping on the foot pedal.

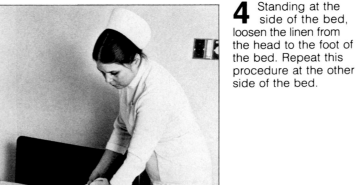

3 Now, remove the pillow from the bed. Slip off the pillowcase, and place the pillow on a chair. Put the pillowcase in the hamper bag.

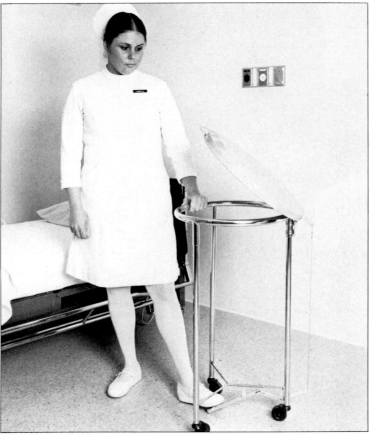

4 Standing at the side of the bed, loosen the linen from the head to the foot of the bed. Repeat this procedure at the other side of the bed.

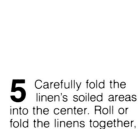

2 Then, fit the hamper bag over the stand's frame, as shown here.

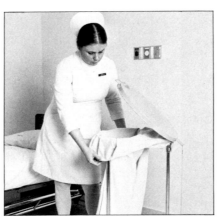

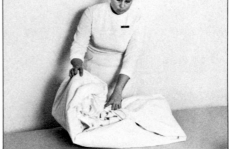

5 Carefully fold the linen's soiled areas into the center. Roll or fold the linens together, as the nurse is doing here.

Then, remove the rolled or folded linens from the bed.

Environmental considerations

How to care for soiled linen continued

6 Holding the linens away from you, open the hamper stand. Place the linens in the hamper bag. Must another bed be changed in the same room? If so, remove the linens from the bed, following steps 4 and 5. Place these linens in the same hamper bag.

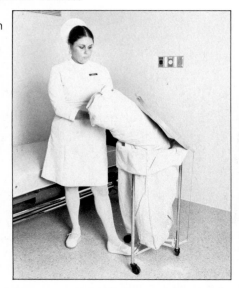

7 Now you're ready to close the hamper bag. To do this, open the hamper stand and lift off the linen bag. Close the linen stand.

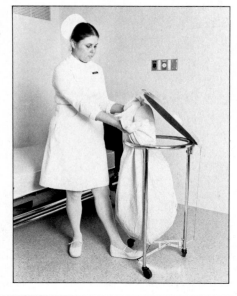

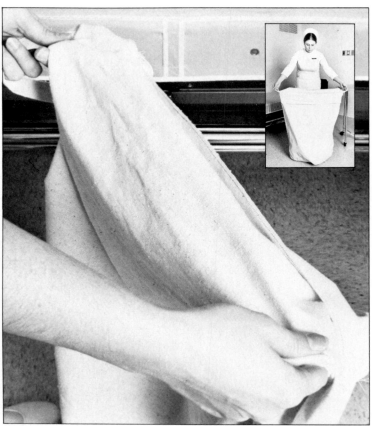

8 Next, pull out the tabs under the flap. That way, the flap will flip over, closing the bag (see inset). This action forces air into the bag, preventing microorganisms from becoming airborne.
Place the hamper bag outside the room.

Then, following your hospital's policy, move on to the next room and repeat this procedure. Or, wash your hands and begin your patient care duties.

When you're completely finished stripping the linens, wash your hands and carry all the hamper bags to the laundry, according to hospital policy. In some hospitals, this responsibility belongs to housekeeping or maintenance personnel.

Dealing with water carafes and ice

In many hospitals, one nursing responsibility is to keep individual patient carafes filled with water and ice. However, water carafes support the growth of some gram-negative organisms. So, to prevent gram-negative organism growth you'll want to care properly for carafes and their contents.

Here are some guidelines to keep in mind:
• Use individual, disposable carafes and cups with lids, whenever possible. Dispose of cups daily. But, if your hospital doesn't use disposable carafes and cups, replace the water glass daily.
• Once each day, wash your patient's carafe with a detergent, following hospital policy. When the patient's discharged, send the carafe to central supply for sterilization, discard it, or send the carafe home with the patient.
• Empty carafes in your unit pantry, not your patient's room.

• Make sure ice is transported in clean, covered containers or plastic bags.
• Check ice storage containers and machines to make sure they're cleaned and disinfected routinely, according to hospital policy.
• Fill carafes in your unit pantry, not your patient's room.
• Use a scoop or tongs when handling ice. Never pick up ice with your hands.
• When not in use, keep ice scoop or tongs in a plastic bag or covered on a clean tray next to the ice bucket or bag. Never place scoop or tongs in the ice bag or bucket.
• Be sure scoop and tongs are washed daily in dishwasher or by hand, following hospital policy.
• Discard any unused ice. Never return unused ice from the patient's water carafe to the storage container.

Cleaning wheelchairs and stretchers

1 *As you know, you'll clean wheelchairs and stretchers weekly, or whenever they become soiled or contaminated. Depending on your hospital's policy, you'll clean wheelchairs and stretchers in the dirty utility room, or other designated area, using a pistol-gripped bottle of germicidal solution. Here's how:*
Begin by slipping a pair of gloves onto your hands.

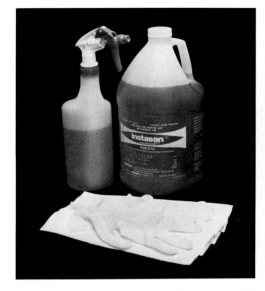

2 To clean a wheelchair, spray all surfaces with the germicidal solution. Use a paper towel to properly distribute the solution.

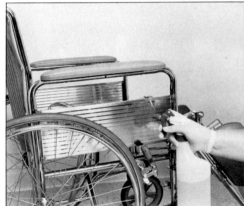

3 Carefully wipe the entire wheelchair, including padding. Then, let the chair dry by exposing it to the air.

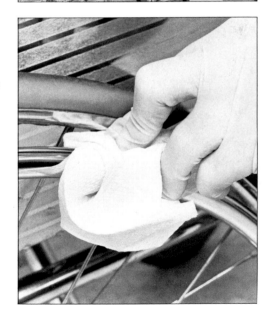

4 Suppose you're preparing to clean a stretcher with germicidal solution and a gauze pad. First, remove the sheet from the stretcher, as the nurse is doing in this photo. Discard the sheet in the laundry hamper.

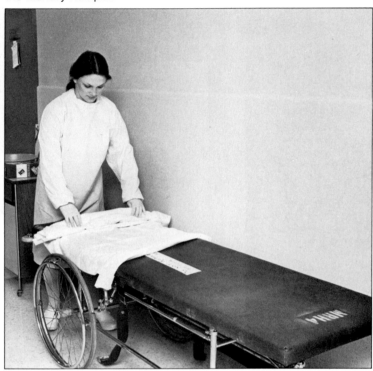

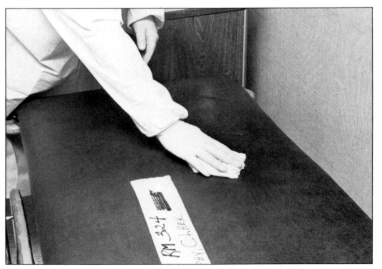

5 Next, moisten the gauze pad in germicidal solution. Wipe the top surface of the stretcher pad with the gauze pad.
Also, clean the stretcher's legs and bottom shelf, if applicable. Expose the stretcher to the air to dry.
Place a clean sheet over the stretcher pad. Finally, remove your gloves.
Note: According to hospital policy, store wheelchairs and stretchers in specified storage areas, never in hallways or patient rooms.

Environmental considerations

Cleaning a thermometer

Anytime you use a thermometer you'll have to make sure it's cared for properly. Why? Because contaminants from excretions, secretions, or the environment create a health hazard for others who use or handle the thermometer. Of course, you'll always follow your hospital's policy, but here are some general thermometer-care guidelines:

• Wash the thermometer holder or container weekly with tincture of green soap. Rinse the holder well with warm, running water and expose it to the air to dry.

• Keep oral and rectal thermometers in separate containers. Label the containers RECTAL thermometers and ORAL thermometers. *Never use an oral thermometer for a rectal temperature, or a rectal thermometer for an oral temperature.*

• Discard thermometer when a patient's discharged from isolation; when he has a known communicable disease requiring isolation (use proper bagging technique); or if the thermometer's cracked.

• Use a disposable thermometer for isolation patients, if possible. Thermometers used in isolation are usually discarded. However, some hospitals clean and disinfect them.

Using a bedside thermometer

1 *Thirty-two-year-old Susan Ewing has been admitted to the medical/surgical unit where you work. She's suffering from a fever of unknown origin. The doctor wants Ms. Ewing's temperature taken every 2 hours for 24 hours. He asks to be called when her temperature spikes above 101.3° F. (38.5° C.). You've decided to use an individual patient bedside thermometer because it reduces the risk of cross-contamination.*

This photostory will show you how to use both an oral and rectal bedside thermometer.

Begin by telling your patient what you're going to do and why. Answer any of her questions. Then, wash your hands with soap and warm, running water. Turn off the faucets with a paper towel to avoid contaminating your hands.

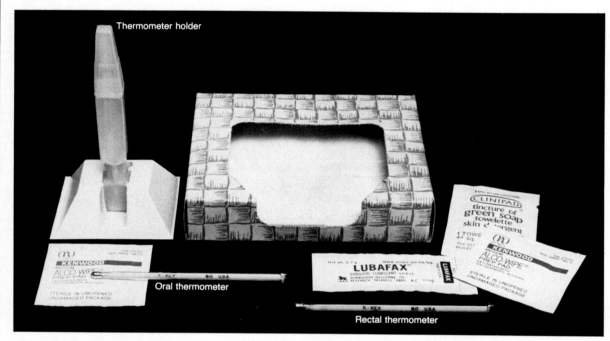

Thermometer holder

Oral thermometer

LUBAFAX

Rectal thermometer

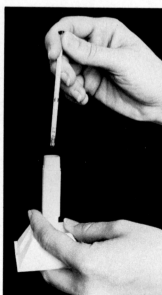

2 Now, remove the thermometer from the holder, as the nurse is doing here. Then, shake it down.

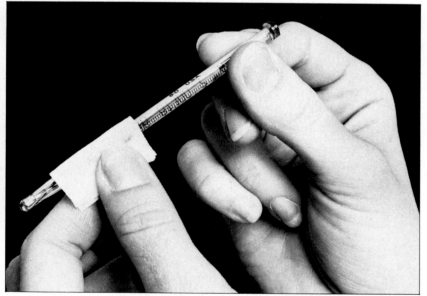

3 Using an alcohol pad, disinfect the thermometer by wiping it from the top end to the bulb. As you do, be sure the pad surrounds the entire thermometer. Discard the pad and rinse the thermometer under cool, running water. Check the reading.

4 Place the thermometer under Ms. Ewing's tongue, as shown here. Warn her not to bite down hard on it. Doing so may crack the thermometer.

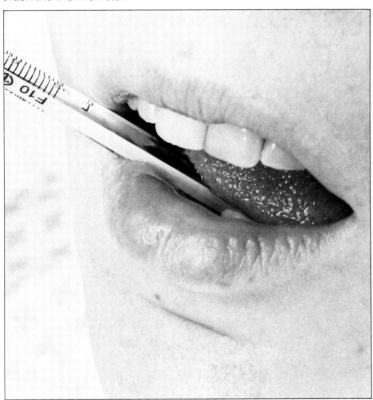

6 Now, here's how to use an individual bedside rectal thermometer. First, shake it down. Then, insert the thermometer into a package of water-soluble lubricant, as shown here. Turn your patient onto her side. Then, carefully insert about 1″ (2.5 cm) of the thermometer into your patient's rectum.

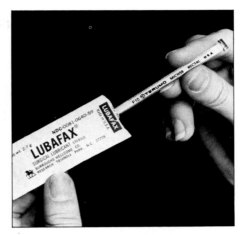

7 When 2 to 4 minutes have passed, remove the thermometer. Use a clean tissue to wipe it from the top end to the bulb. Read the thermometer.
Then, clean the thermometer from the top end to the bulb with tincture of green soap wipe and cold, running water. Discard the wipe.

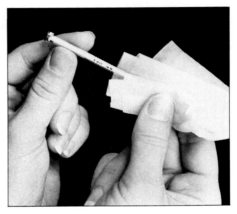

5 After 8 or 9 minutes, remove the thermometer from your patient's mouth. Using a clean tissue, remove saliva by wiping the thermometer from the top end to the bulb, as the nurse is doing here. *Remember:* Always wipe a thermometer from the cleanest to the most contaminated end. Then, discard the tissue into the wastebasket and read the thermometer.
Next, use a new alcohol pad to wipe the thermometer from the top end to the bulb. Discard the pad into the wastebasket. Place the thermometer in its holder. Remember, dry storage prevents organism growth.

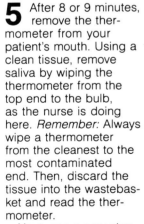

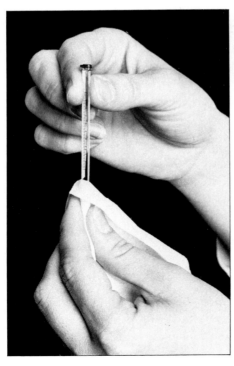

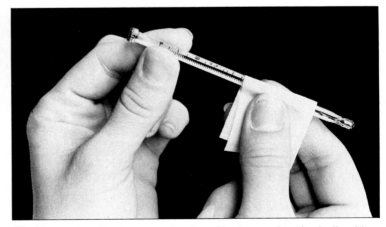

8 Next, wipe the thermometer from the top end to the bulb with an alcohol pad. Place the rectal thermometer in its dry holder. Wash your hands with soap and water. Remember to turn off the faucets with a paper towel.
Finally, document the procedure in your nurses' notes. Also record Ms. Ewing's temperature, the date, and time on her temperature chart.
Then, when she's discharged, send the thermometer home with her, clean and disinfect it, or discard it, according to hospital policy.

Environmental considerations

Using a Temp-Away™ sheath

1 *In this photostory, we'll show you how to use a Temp-Away oral thermometer sheath for an individual patient thermometer.*

Begin by telling your patient what you're going to do. Then, wash your hands with soap and warm, running water. Remove the thermometer from the covered container and shake it down.

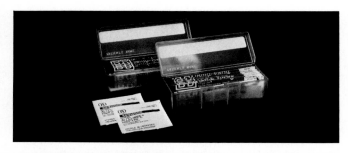

2 Now, slip the thermometer into the paper-covered Temp-Away sheath. Twist the paper covering on the dotted line, as shown here. Remember, if you're using a rectal thermometer, use a prelubricated Temp-Away sheath.

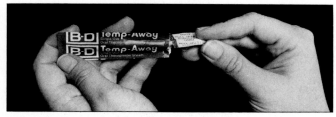

3 Gently, but firmly, pull off the sheath's paper cover. Expect a plastic sheath to encase the thermometer. If the thermometer's not encased in plastic, discard the sheath and obtain a new one. Start the procedure again.

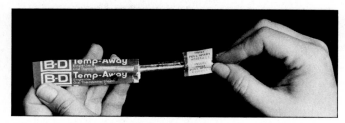

4 Next, place the thermometer under your patient's tongue. Wait 8 to 9 minutes. Then, remove the thermometer from your patient's mouth. Pull the sheath's top tab downward. The sheath will invert as it's removed, enclosing secretions and bacteria. Discard the sheath in a covered waste receptacle. Read the thermometer.

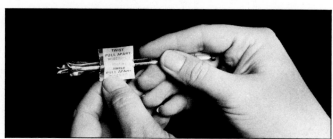

5 Shake down the thermometer again. Wipe the thermometer from the top end to the bulb with an alcohol pad. Discard the pad.

Return the thermometer to its covered container. Then, wash your hands. Finally, document the procedure in your notes, and record on the patient's temperature chart his temperature, and the date and time.

Remember, any tear in the thermometer's sheath will allow microorganisms from your patient's mouth to contaminate the thermometer. So, when your patient's discharged, clean and disinfect the thermometer, discard it, or send it home with him, following hospital policy.

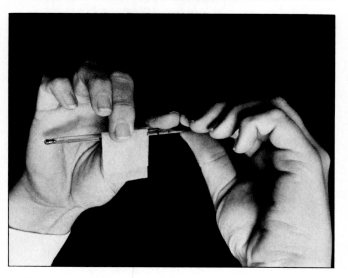

How to use an electronic thermometer

1 *Follow these steps carefully to use an IVAC® electronic rectal thermometer.*

First wash your hands with soap and water. To avoid contamination, use a paper towel to turn off the faucets. Then, hang the IVAC thermometer around your neck (see inset).

2 As you explain the procedure to your patient, grasp the thermometer's probe by the collar. Remove the rectal probe from the face of the thermometer (see photo). This automatically turns on the thermometer, displaying a digital temperature reading of 94° F.

3 Now, press the probe firmly into a probe cover. Take care not to touch the top of the probe, which serves as the ejection button.

Note: The rectal probe does not require lubrication.

Continue to hold the probe's collar, as you insert about 1″ (2.5 cm) of the probe's tip into your patient's rectum. Hold the probe steady and tilt it slightly to ensure proper body tissue contact. When you hear a beep and see the red light go on, remove the probe from your patient's rectum. Note the temperature reading. Is the probe cover soiled? Wrap tissues around it and proceed.

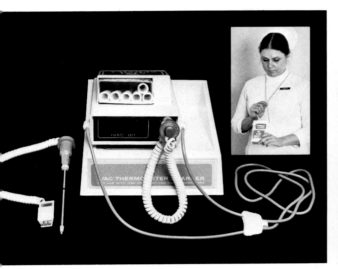

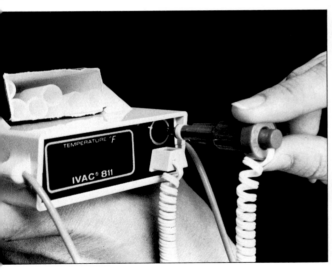

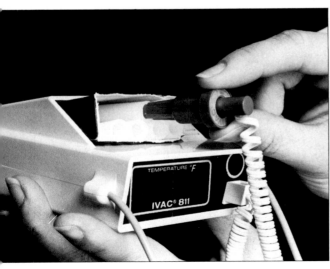

4 Now you're ready to remove the cover from the probe. To do this, hold the probe collar between your index and middle fingers. Now, with your thumb, press the top of the probe, as the nurse is doing here. The probe cover will pop off. Discard the probe cover in a covered trash receptacle.

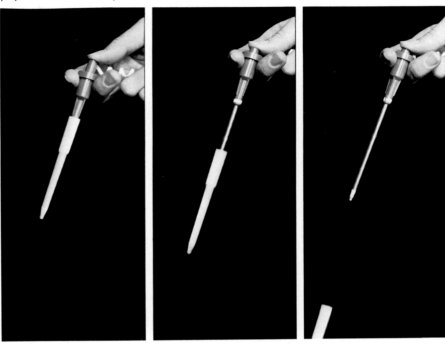

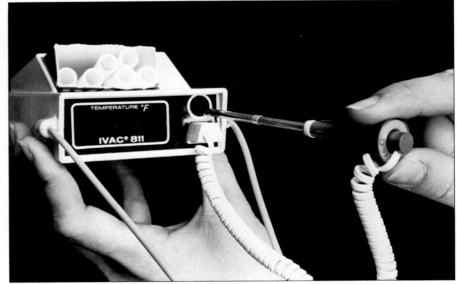

5 Return the probe to the face of the thermometer. Doing so will automatically turn off and reset the thermometer.

Finally, wash your hands, and document the procedure in your nurses' notes. Be sure to record the patient's temperature, the date, and time on his temperature chart.

Note: When not in use, store the thermometer in the self-charging base. Routinely clean the thermometer with a disinfectant/detergent solution, or have it gas sterilized, following your hospital's and the manufacturer's policy.

Environmental considerations

How to use a Tempa-Dot™ single-use strip thermometer

1 *We've told you how to use an individual bedside thermometer, a thermometer sheath, and an electronic thermometer. But do you know how to properly use a disposable Tempa-Dot single-use oral thermometer? Read these guidelines to refresh your memory.*

Begin by washing your hands with soap and warm, running water. Remember to turn off the faucets with a paper towel.

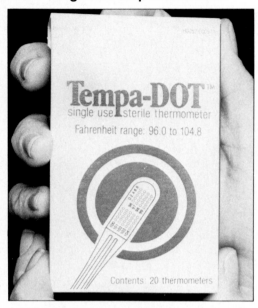

2 Then, carefully remove the thermometer strip from the package. To do this, bend the package forward and backward at the dotted line, as the nurse is doing in the inset.

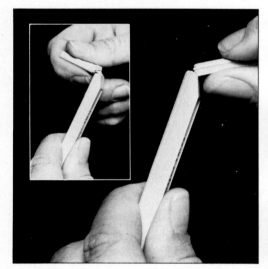

3 As you pull the thermometer out of the package, take care not to touch the dotted area, which is the sensor matrix.

Note: Always pull the thermometer straight out of the package. Any twisting or side-to-side movement may tear the thermometer. Discard the package in a covered waste receptacle.

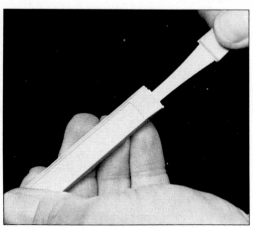

4 Now, explain the procedure to your patient as you position the thermometer diagonally under his tongue. Instruct your patient to close his mouth. Take care to position the thermometer carefully to avoid paper cuts.

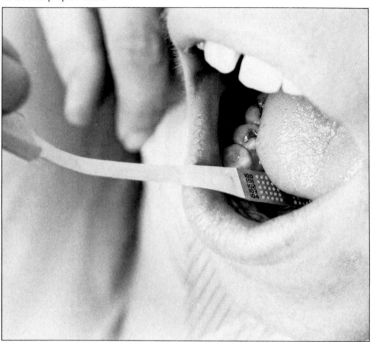

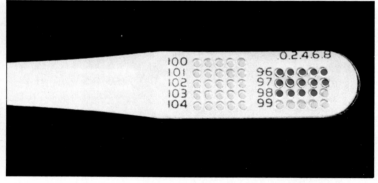

5 After about 1 minute, remove the Tempa-Dot thermometer from your patient's mouth. Wait 5 seconds before reading the thermometer. Doing so allows the last few dots to register.

The last dot that changes from white to green indicates the temperature.

Finally, discard the thermometer in the covered waste receptacle. Wash your hands and document the procedure.

But what if the thermometer doesn't register a temperature? Place it back under your patient's tongue for 45 seconds. Suppose the thermometer still doesn't register a temperature. Discard the thermometer, and obtain a new one. Then, follow the procedure above.

Note: Always store Tempa-Dot single-use thermometers in a cool area, preferably less than 86° F. (30° C.). Avoid exposing them to direct sunlight, because heat may cause the thermometer to register temperature.

Housekeeping: What to know

You're probably aware of how efficient housekeeping relates to infection control. The health of everyone in the hospital, including visitors, is affected by how well cleaning duties are performed during and after a patient's hospital stay (concurrent and terminal cleaning). Do you know what housekeeping's basic responsibilities are? If you're unsure, read on:

• *Carpeted floors* should be vacuumed daily with equipment that doesn't stir up microorganisms.

Note: Carpeted floors are not recommended in patient-care areas.

• *Uncarpeted open areas* should be cleaned with a wet-vacuum machine or wet mop. Dry mopping is unacceptable. The cleaning solution should be prepared daily to prevent contamination. Never add fresh solution to solution prepared earlier.

• *Walls and furniture* may be cleaned with wet cloths and mops, using a germicidal solution.

• *Beds and mattresses* should be cleaned with fresh disinfectant solution and a cleaning cloth during the terminal cleaning process.

• *Isolation rooms* should be cleaned the same way as any other area. But keep the cleaning materials and solution used for this chore in the isolation room; never allow them to be used in other areas of the hospital. After terminal cleaning, disposable cleaning materials should be discarded, according to hospital policy. Double bag mop heads and send to the central supply department. Also, cleaning personnel should wear appropriate isolation garb while cleaning the isolation room.

• *Bathrooms* should be cleaned last. Why? Because toilets and sinks may be contaminated. Never use a bathroom cleaning cloth or toilet-bowl brush to clean any other area in the room or hospital.

Here are some more reminders:

• Mop heads and dusters should be laundered daily.

• Wet mops and sponges should be stored dry in the janitor's closet. Make sure mops and sponges aren't stored in water.

• Cleaning buckets must be emptied before storing.

• Prepare and use all cleaning solutions according to manufacturer's instructions.

Teaching your patient about infection

Seven hospital employees, including your patient, 19-year-old X-ray technician Bridget Norwood, have *salmonella* infections. After taking an accurate history, you find that all seven employees ate the hospital cafeteria's chicken salad approximately 36 hours ago. Apparently, the chicken salad was spoiled. What do you do?

Report the incident to your hospital's infection-control practitioner. Then, reassure Bridget. Find out how much she knows about *salmonella*. Don't assume someone has already explained *salmonella* to her. Even if they have, she may have been too sick or too frightened to understand what was being explained. Encourage her to ask any questions. Then, answer them as honestly and completely as possible.

Now, study the dialogue that follows. It'll help you anticipate questions or misconceptions your patient may have.

Patient's question: Why did I get sick from the chicken salad?
Your answer: That's difficult to say. The chicken may have been contaminated with *salmonella* organisms before it was cooked. Or, the chicken salad may have been contaminated during or after preparation.

Patient's question: How did the chicken salad become spoiled?
Your answer: Poultry can become contaminated with *salmonella* organisms before it is cooked. These organisms come from the poultry feed. However, thorough cooking destroys *salmonella*. But improper cooking, handling, or storing allows *salmonella* organisms to multiply and cause an infection after you've eaten.

Patient's question: How can I avoid getting *salmonella* or other similiar infections again?
Your answer: Use your common sense. Whenever or wherever you dine, closely inspect the drinking glasses, plates, utensils, and your food. If the glasses, plates, or utensils look soiled, ask for new ones. And, if the food looks strange, has an unfamiliar odor, or doesn't taste right, send it back to the kitchen.

When grocery shopping, always check the expiration date on food, dairy, refrigerated, or frozen products. If the date is past due or the product is opened, damaged, or has thawed, don't buy the item, regardless of the price. In addition, always put refrigerated or frozen products in your shopping cart last. That way these products will stay refrigerated or frozen up to the time you check out of the store.

Take your time when purchasing meat, poultry, or fish. If any of these products appears discolored or smells unpleasant, don't buy it, no matter what the salesperson tells you.

Recheck the expiration date on packaged food before preparing the item. If the expiration date has passed, throw out the product. The health risk is never worth the product's cost.

Always wash your hands before preparing any food product. And remember to cook pork, poultry, and fish thoroughly. When not cooked thoroughly, the chance of microorganism growth increases, causing these products to spoil more rapidly.

Patient's question: Will a dishwasher help prevent food-associated infections?
Your answer: Yes, because water in a dishwasher reaches the dishes at a higher temperature than the water from your kitchen faucet. So, dishwashers filled with the proper amount of detergent kill more microorganisms on the dishes.

But, if you don't have a dishwasher, use detergent and warm water to wash your dishes. Detergent kills more microorganisms than soap. Rinse dishes with hot water. And remember, letting your dishes dry by exposing them to the air is better than drying them with a dish towel. Why? Because a dish towel can spread infection (or microorganisms) from one dish, utensil, or glass to another.

Environmental considerations

Preventing food-associated infections: Some tips

Improperly prepared, packaged, or covered food can be a potential infection source. While you won't be around to monitor every bit of food or drink your patient consumes, you can ask for his cooperation. Also, ask for the cooperation of his family and friends.

Try to discourage your patient's family and friends from bringing food from outside sources, unless his condition would deteriorate without it.

Explain the importance of proper food handling and packaging in reducing infection. Stress that a food-associated infection may lengthen the patient's hospital stay.

But, no matter how much teaching you do, your patient may receive food from outside sources. If he does, keep these important guidelines in mind:
• Make sure all food is in a closed container—either plastic or metal. Fruit may be placed in a plastic bag.
• Label all stored food containers with your patient's name, room number, and the date.
• Never store any food for more than a week.
• Offer to store perishable food in your unit's refrigerator. Routinely remind him that the food is still there.
• Don't keep dairy products beyond the expiration date on the carton.
• Check all perishable food closely before serving to your patient.
• Warn your patient not to save partially eaten food and drinks; for example, candy bars and milkshakes.
• Discard all uneaten food in the proper trash receptacle, following your hospital's policy. Usually, at least one receptacle on each unit is designated for this purpose. *Never* place uneaten perishable food in a bedside wastebasket.

Nurses' guide to reportable diseases

Confidential reporting form

Category I - Individual case report of disease

Patient's name		Sex	Birth date

Address	Zip code	County	Telephone #

Race		Died	Date of report
☐ Bl ☐ W ☐ Oriental ☐ Other			

Occupation	Work place or school (name)	Occupational disease?

Disease or suspected disease (If V.D. or T.B. complete below)   Date

If viral hepatitis serum positive for HBsAg   Suspected source
☐ Yes   ☐ No   ☐ Not tested

Hospital name   ☐ Outpatient   ☐ Inpatient   Date admitted

Pertinent laboratory data and comments

Category II - Report by number of cases only

☐ Chicken pox   ☐ Group A beta-   ☐ Other (specify)
                         hemolytic streptococ-   _____
                         cal infections, including
☐ Influenza   scarlet fever   Date

Doctor's name   Address   Telephone #

Venereal disease
Syphilis
☐ Primary ☐ Secondary ☐ Early latent (less than 1 yr.) ☐ Congenital
☐ Other stages (specify)
Gonorrhea
☐ Uncomplicated ☐ Pelvic inflammatory disease ☐ Ophthalmia
☐ Other complications (specify)
Other venereal diseases (specify)

Specify lab test				Treatment given	
Date	Test	Results	Date	Drug	Dosage

Tuberculosis disease
Most significant site of disease
☐ Pulmonary ☐ Pleural ☐ Peritoneal ☐ Meningeal ☐ Lymphatic
☐ Bone joint ☐ G/U ☐ Miliary ☐ Other (specify)
Other sites involved (specify)

Supporting bacteriologic histologic evidence

	Pos.	Neg.	Pending	Not done	Specimen
Smear					Sputum
Culture					Other
Histology					

Chemotherapy   Current prescription   Date started

X-ray
☐ Not done ☐ Normal ☐ Abnormal noncavitary ☐ Cavitary
Previous prescription for tuberculosis disease
☐ Yes   ☐ No   ☐ Positive
Tuberculin test
☐ Not done   ☐ Negative   ☐ Positive
Additional information

Reportable diseases and conditions are usually separated into two categories: those that you'll report individually on the day of diagnosis, or when the diagnosis is suspected; and those that you'll report by the number of cases per week. Fast, accurate reporting helps community health officials identify and control possible infection sources, and possibly avoid epidemic conditions.

Of course, reporting procedures differ from area to area. However, in most cases you'll telephone the information directly to community health officials. Then, you'll fill out a report, like the one at left. Mail the report to community health officials, depending on your hospital's policy. But remember, use the information below only as a guide. Always follow your hospital's policy.

Category I
The diseases and conditions that follow must be reported as soon as they're diagnosed, or when the diagnosis is suspected. When reporting these diseases, include the patient's name, date, sex, and address. If possible, include his telephone number.
• amebiasis
• animal bites
• anthrax (inhalation or cutaneous)
• botulism
• brucellosis
• cholera
• diphtheria (pharyngeal or cutaneous)
• encephalitis; primary (specific etiology); post infectious
• food-poisoning outbreaks
• gastroenteritis (institutional outbreaks only)
• Guillain-Barré syndrome
• hepatitis type A (HBsAg negative); specify suspected source, such as water or shellfish
• hepatitis type B (HBsAg positive); specify suspected source, such as needles or blood products

- hepatitis type non-A, non-B; specify suspected source, such as needles or blood transfusions
- Legionnaires' disease
- leprosy
- leptospirosis
- malaria
- meningitis (specify etiology)
- meningococcal disease
- mumps
- occupational or industrial diseases, such as chronic or acute illnesses that may be induced by the patient's employment environment
- pertussis
- plague (pneumonic or bubonic)
- poisoning or adverse reactions from drugs or other toxic agents
- psittacosis
- rabies (human)
- post-exposure rabies prophylaxis
- Reye's syndrome
- Rocky Mountain spotted fever
- rubella (confirmation by inhibition test recommended)
- rubella syndrome (congenital)
- rubeola
- salmonellosis
- shigellosis
- smallpox
- staphylococcal infections (newborn infants only)
- tetanus
- trichinosis
- tuberculosis (complete the entire form)
- tularemia
- typhoid fever
- typhus
- venereal disease (complete the entire form)
- yellow fever.

Category II
The diseases listed below are reported by the number of cases a week. You don't need the name of the patient to file your report.
- chicken pox
- Group A beta-hemolytic streptococcal infections, including scarlet fever
- influenza

Understanding employee health exams

Whether you work in a hospital, nursing home, or clinic, you probably know something about employee health exams. But, do you know why these exams are so important? For starters, employee health screening helps detect conditions dangerous to you, your coworkers, potential employees, and patients. In most cases, health screening is divided into two parts: preemployment health exams and routine health exams.

Before we discuss routine health exams, let's review the preemployment health exam. As you know, most hospitals avoid the expense of obtaining complete medical histories and physical exams by screening only for specific diseases.

Important: A preemployment health exam does not negate your need for an annual health examination.

Here's what is usually required on a preemployment health exam:
- history of any communicable diseases, such as measles, mumps, hepatitis, tuberculosis; or a history of diarrhea, chronic skin conditions or infections
- venereal disease research laboratory (VDRL) test to identify secondary syphilis. This, as you know, is a blood test.
- tuberculin test (purified protein derivative) to identify tuberculosis. If you have a history of a positive reaction, you may be able to have this test waived. But, you'll need written or oral communication from the previous testing area to your health-care facility. If you can't obtain this data, you'll be retested.

Suppose the tuberculin test is positive. Then, you'll need a chest X-ray, although chest X-rays are contraindicated if you're pregnant.
- color-blindness test for laboratory personnel
- serum antibody titer for females of childbearing age; as well as for pediatric, nursery, and obstetric personnel to identify rubella and rubeola susceptibility

- mumps vaccine for obstetrics, nursery, and pediatric personnel who haven't had the disease
- diphtheria and tetanus vaccines if you haven't been vaccinated, or if it has been 10 years since your last booster
- an electrocardiogram (EKG), if you're over 40.

Usually, the procedure for routine or follow-up health exams depends on the hospital unit where you work. But here are some general guidelines:
- Do you work in the hemodialysis or peritoneal dialysis unit? If so, you'll need a monthly blood test for hepatitis B surface antigen (HB_sAg) and serum glutamic-oxaloacetic transaminase (SGOT). If the HB_sAg level is positive and reconfirmed on a second test, you'll need an SGOT and a serum glutamic-pyruvic transaminase (SGPT) test to determine liver function. You'll also be checked for anti-HB_s levels. If the SGOT and SGPT results are normal, you'll probably be allowed to return to work. However, you may be assigned to care for patients who also have HB_sAg positive levels. When the SGOT and SGPT results are abnormal, you'll be off work until the levels return to normal or additional studies show that you don't have active viral hepatitis B.
- If you work in an obstetrics unit, you'll need an annual VDRL.
- If you work in a nursing unit, clinic, admissions department, respiratory therapy or microbiology department, and have had a negative tuberculin reaction, you'll need a tuberculin test once every 6 months. If you work in any other area and have had a negative reaction, you'll need the test repeated annually.
- If you've had a positive chest X-ray, you'll need a repeat chest X-ray every year.

Remember, if you can prove that you've had any of the tests mentioned above within the past year, you may not need them repeated. But, you must provide your hospital with a record of the test performed, doctor's name, and results.

Learning about the infection-control practitioner: Duties and responsibilities

You may know the name of the infection-control practitioner in your hospital. But do you know what she does? An infection-control practitioner is responsible for designing and implementing an infection-control program that meets the specific needs of the institution.

About three quarters of all infection-control practitioners are registered nurses. Why? Because the responsibilities of the infection-control practitioner require good knowledge of nursing skills and hospital services.

The infection-control practitioner's day-to-day responsibilities cover many areas of the hospital. For starters, she works with the infection-control committee to establish and review isolation policies and procedures. She also organizes hospital inservices to keep hospital personnel up to date

on isolation precautions and infection-control procedures. She works with hospital staff members to help identify, treat, and prevent nosocomial infections. She also may oversee the employee-health program, or act as a consultant. In addition, the infection-control practitioner reviews patient records and culture- and sensitivity-test results to determine if the proper antibiotics and treatments have been administered. In cases where a microorganism appears resistant to the administered antibiotic, she may make specific recommendations to the doctor.

The responsibilities of an infection-control practitioner vary from hospital to hospital. But all infection-control practitioners share one common goal: minimize the spread of infection among patients, hospital personnel, and visitors.

Environmental considerations

Protecting employees from infection

While emptying a trash receptacle, Tom Brady, a member of the house-keeping staff, accidentally sticks his finger with a needle that was disposed of improperly. After some careful checking, you discover that the needle came from an intravenous line of a patient with hepatitis B.

In most hospitals, your next step is to notify the doctor who supervises employee-health matters. He'll probably do one of two things: arrange to examine Mr. Brady as soon as possible, or advise Mr. Brady to see his family doctor.

Following Mr. Brady's examination, the decision for prophylactic therapy will be based on:
• potential infectiousness of the patient
• type and duration of contact
• results of lab tests
• host susceptibility.

In Mr. Brady's case, his family doctor ordered hyperimmune serum globulin, human, administered I.M. immediately. He instructed Mr. Brady to return in 28 to 30 days for a repeat dose.

Remember: Opinions on appropriate prophylactic therapy differ. Always follow your hospital's established policy.

Administering a tuberculin test

1 *Is tuberculin skin testing part of your hospital's preemployment health screening? If your hospital uses the tuberculin purified protein derivative (PPD) intradermal skin test, proceed as follows:*

First, assemble the equipment you'll need: tuberculin purified protein derivative (PPD) serum, 1 cc 25G tuberculin syringe with needle, and several alcohol prep pads. You may also need a 2"x2" sterile gauze pad.

The nurse in this photostory will be using Aplisol tuberculin test serum.

Wash your hands with soap and warm water, and dry them with a paper towel. Use a paper towel to turn off the faucets.

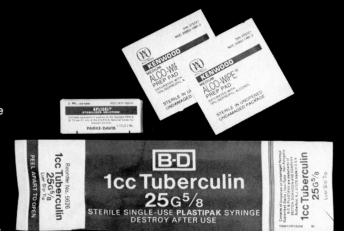

2 Check the Aplisol vial to make sure it's not outdated or contaminated. If the serum is okay, draw it up into the syringe. Then, cap the syringe.

Explain the test procedure to your patient. Ask her about any allergies or past skin-test reactions. If she's had a positive tuberculin reaction, notify the doctor. He may choose another type of tuberculin test.

Position your patient's ventral forearm on a flat surface to expose it. Slightly flex her elbow.

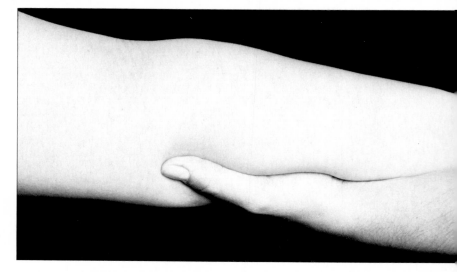

3 Now you're ready to select an injection site. To do this, locate your patient's antecubital space. Then, measure about 2" to 3" (5.1 to 7.6 cm) from the antecubital space toward the patient's hand. You should be about 4" to 5" (10.2 to 12.7 cm) away from the wrist. Avoid choosing a skin area with hair or blemishes.

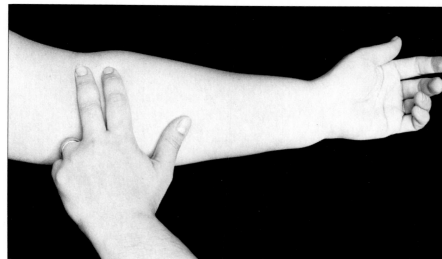

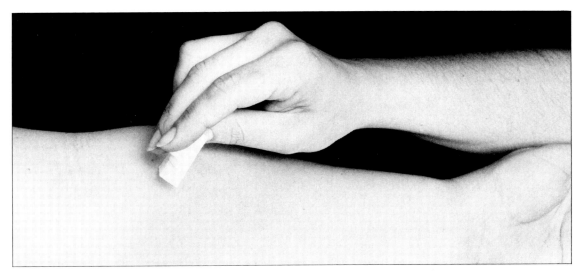

4 Next, clean your patient's skin thoroughly with an alcohol prep pad. To do this, begin at the center of the injection site and move outward in a circular motion. Never clean the skin with a disinfectant, such as Betadine, which will discolor the injection area. Also, avoid rubbing the skin vigorously with the alcohol prep pad. Either action may interfere with accurate test results. Dry the skin by exposing it to air.

Pull the skin taut on the patient's forearm. Do this by holding your patient's forearm in one hand and stretching her skin with your thumb.

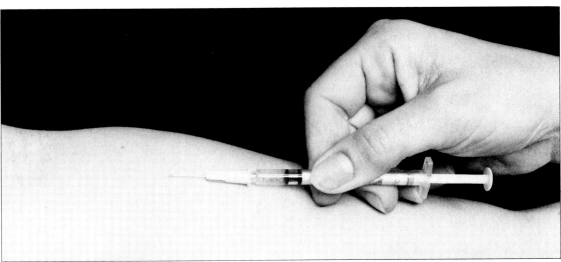

5 Now, with your other hand, uncap the syringe. Expel any air in the syringe. Hold the syringe between your thumb and forefinger, as shown here.

Position the syringe so that the needle is almost flat against the patient's skin. Make sure the needle bevel is up.

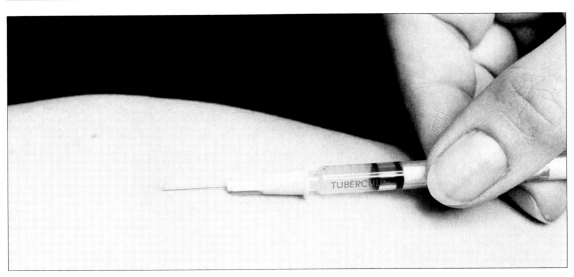

6 Insert the needle by pressing against the skin until you meet resistance. Then, advance the needle through the epidermis, so the point of the needle is visible through the skin. Stop when the needle's resting ⅛″ (3 mm) below the skin surface, between the epidermis and dermal layers.

Environmental considerations

Administering a tuberculin test continued

7 Inject the serum as slowly and gently as possible. Expect to feel some resistance. If the needle moves too freely, you've inserted it too deeply. Withdraw it slightly and try again. When you've finished injecting the medication, leave the needle in place momentarily. Watch for the appearance of a small, white blister or wheal (about 6 mm in diameter).

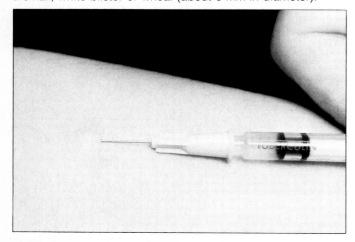

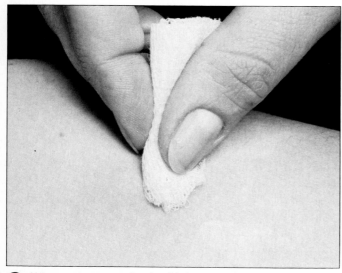

8 When you see a wheal, withdraw the needle, and apply gentle pressure to the site. Don't massage the site, because doing so may interfere with the test results.

Next, document in your notes the name of the test given, dosage, time, date, and patient's name. If the patient has an allergic reaction within 30 minutes, notify the doctor. He may order 1:1,000 epinephrine administered immediately.

Tell your patient to return in 48 to 72 hours so you can read the test results. When your patient returns, carefully examine the test site. Look for vesicle formation and measure the extent of induration in millimeters. Also measure erythema, if present. However, erythema with hardening is not significant. If the induration is less than 2 mm without vesiculation, the test is negative. But, if you see vesiculation, the test is positive. Your patient may have tuberculosis.

Document the test results in your nurses' notes.

Infectious diseases: When to stay home

You probably know how to identify the signs and symptoms of most infectious diseases and conditions. But when you have an infectious disease or condition, do you know how long to stay off the job? Or when you can continue working?

The chart below gives you some sample guidelines. But remember, always follow your hospital's policy.

Condition or disease	Work status	Work return
Active tuberculosis	Off	May return when condition's being treated with appropriate drug therapy, and sputum smears have been negative for 2 weeks.
Positive purified protein derivative reaction	May work	Contact employee-health service for evaluation and follow-up.
Chicken pox (varicella)	Off	May return 7 days after first eruption.
Conjunctivitis, viral	May work	Transfer to nondirect patient care.
Diarrhea, shigella, salmonella	Varies	Check with employee-health committee. Decision depends on culture results and severity of signs and symptoms.
Draining wounds (Staphylococcus aureus, abscess, laceration)	Off	May return when drainage stops.
Gonorrhea	May work	None
Hepatitis A	Off	Need doctor's written approval before returning to work.
Hepatitis B	Off	Need doctor's written approval before returning to work.
Herpes simplex	May work	Check with employee-health committee. Decision depends on hospital unit.
Herpes zoster	May work	Transfer to nondirect patient care.
Impetigo	May work	Transfer to nondirect patient care unit until crusts heal.
Mononucleosis	Off	Check with your doctor. He'll decide when you may return to work.
Pediculosis (lice)	Off	May return when condition's being treated.
Rubella (German measles)	Off	May return when rash disappears; usually off at least 5 days.
Rubeola (measles)	Off	May return when rash disappears; usually off at least 4 days.
Scabies	Off	May return when condition's being treated.
Streptococcus infections	Off	May return 24 hours after effective therapy.
Upper respiratory infections and influenza	Varies	Check with employee-health committee. Decision depends on hospital unit where you work.

Cleaning, disinfecting, and sterilizing

No doubt you're aware how cleaning, disinfecting, and sterilizing procedures help prevent infection. You probably perform some of these procedures as part of your nursing routine.

But, how familiar are you with specific techniques? For example, do you know how to clean a soiled article? Or wrap a linen pack for sterilization?

If you're uncertain, read the following section. We'll show you how to perform these procedures as well as review basic hand-washing technique. In addition, we'll explain which antiseptics prove most effective against specific organisms, how disinfectants differ, and why one sterilization method may be better than another.

Reviewing basic terms

To refresh your memory on disinfecting and sterilizing procedures, let's review some basic terms.

Antiseptic: An agent which stops or inhibits, but does not necessarily kill, microorganisms contaminating the skin or other tissues

Asepsis: Absence of disease-producing microorganisms

Bactericidal: An agent that destroys bacteria present on a surface, but not their spores

Bacteriostatic: An agent that inhibits, but does not necessarily kill, bacterial growth on a surface

Cleaning: Removing dirt and debris from a surface

Contamination: Presence of disease-producing microorganisms on an object

Cross-contamination: Transmission of disease-producing microorganisms from one object to another

Decontamination: Removal of disease-producing microorganisms from an object

Disinfection: The process of destroying disease-producing microorganisms, but not their spores, on inanimate objects

Germicidal: An agent that destroys germs on a surface

Liquid sterilization: Germicidal process of destroying and eliminating all microorganisms and their products over an extended time period. Used on articles that can be damaged by heat.

Spores: Reproductive part of a specific microorganism, such as those of a protozoan, fungus, or bacterium

Sterile: Absence of all living microorganisms, including spores, from a surface

Sterilization: Process of destroying and eliminating all microorganisms and their products

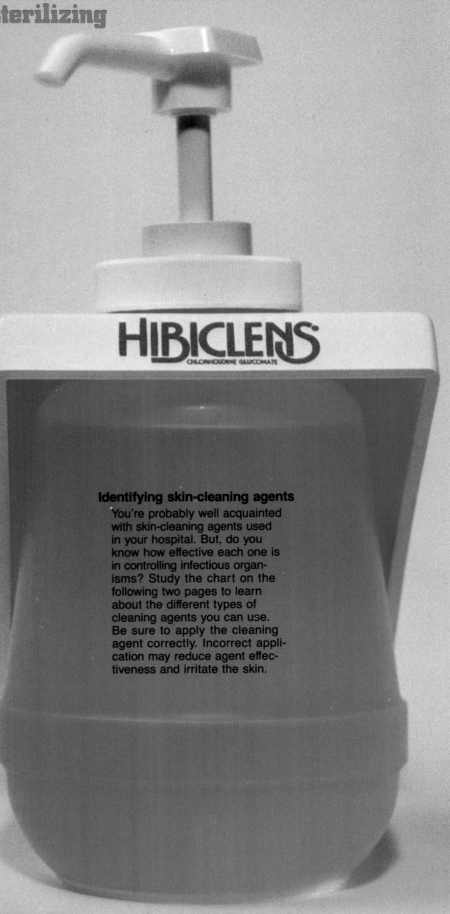

Identifying skin-cleaning agents

You're probably well acquainted with skin-cleaning agents used in your hospital. But, do you know how effective each one is in controlling infectious organisms? Study the chart on the following two pages to learn about the different types of cleaning agents you can use. Be sure to apply the cleaning agent correctly. Incorrect application may reduce agent effectiveness and irritate the skin.

Cleaning, disinfecting, and sterilizing

Identifying skin-cleaning agents continued

Bar soap

Examples
- Ivory®
- Safeguard®

Use
- Helps remove organisms but doesn't kill them.

Nursing considerations
- After using, store agent on drainable rack. Clean rack regularly.
- For maximum effectiveness, get a new supply when agent is half gone.

Chlorhexidine gluconate

Examples
- Hibiclens®
- Hibistat™
- Hibitane®

Use
- Destroys gram-positive and gram-negative organisms, fungi, and viruses.

Nursing considerations
- Use sparingly. Agent does not produce suds.
- Do not use with alcohol or normal saline solution.
- Rinse thoroughly after use.
- If used repeatedly, effectiveness increases.

Dry soap

Examples
- Boraxo®
- Granules or Pre-Op® soap tissues

Use
- Helps remove organisms but doesn't kill them.

Nursing considerations
- Keep dispenser dry to prevent it from clogging.
- After applying, scrub hands about 15 seconds to dissolve agent.

Foaming alcohol

Example
- Alcare™

Use
- Destroys gram-positive and gram-negative organisms and fungi.

Nursing considerations
- Can be used for cleaning when water is unavailable.
- Use sufficient amount of foam to keep hands moist for 30 to 60 seconds.
- Can be given to patients for their personal use.

Hexachlorophene

Examples
- pHisoHex®
- Turgex®

Use
- Destroys gram-positive organisms.

Nursing considerations
- Try to avoid frequent use. Agent may irritate skin and lead to serious neurotoxic effects. Always rinse skin thoroughly after use.

Liquid soap without antiseptic

Examples
- Safe 'n Sure® lotion soap
- Vestal lotion soap
- Tincture of green soap

Use
- Helps remove organisms but doesn't kill them.

Nursing considerations
- To help prevent the growth of microorganisms, regularly empty, clean, and refill dispenser, following your hospital's policy.

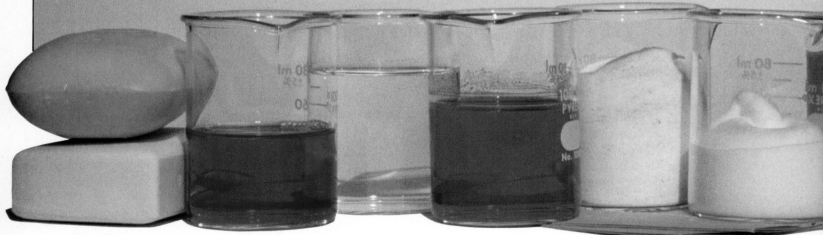

Safeguard®
Ivory®   Hibiclens®   Hibistat™   Hibitane®   Boraxo®   Pre-Op soap tissues®   Alcare™

Iodine

Example
• Tincture of iodine

Use
• Destroys gram-positive and gram-negative organisms, *Mycobacterium tuberculosis*, spores, and fungi.

Nursing considerations
• Do not use if iodine allergy exists.
• Rinse treated area with alcohol about 30 seconds after applying agent. May stain skin or cause irritation and burning. Agent also stains fabrics.
• Expose treated area to air. Do not bandage.

Povidone-iodine

Examples
• Betadine®
• Povadyne® cleansing bar
• Surgi-scrub™ III
• Acu-Dyne® skin cleanser

Use
• Destroys gram-positive and gram-negative organisms, viruses, and fungi.

Nursing considerations
• After applying, rinse with water.
• If using Betadine solution, keep on skin; rinsing reduces effectiveness. However, if you must see vein, remove agent with alcohol.
• Avoid frequent use. Agent may irritate skin. May cause skin burns, if iodine allergic.

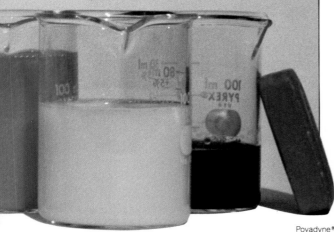

Turgex®   Safe 'n Sure lotion soap®   Tincture of iodine   Povadyne® cleansing bar

Reviewing basic hand-washing techniques

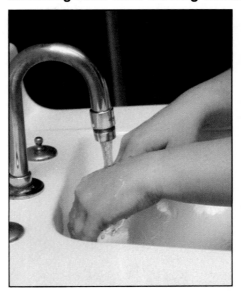

1 *How often do you wash your hands? If you're like most nurses, you will no doubt answer "Frequently!" But, according to infection-control standards, probably not frequently enough.*

As you know, hand washing provides one of the best ways to prevent and control infections. Follow these steps to refresh your memory on basic technique:

First, remove all rings except a plain wedding band, if you're wearing one. Then, wet your hands under warm, running water.

Note: The nurse in this photostory is using a sink with foot controls for soap and water. Always use foot or knee controls for soap and water in any high-risk area.

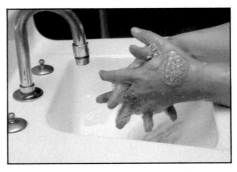

2 Apply the proper amount of soap or antiseptic cleaning agent, such as Acu-Dyne. Work up a lather by vigorously rubbing your hands together, fingers intertwined. Doing so creates friction, which loosens dirt and organisms. If necessary, use a scrub brush. Scrub for at least 15 seconds over every part of your hands, including between your fingers, knuckles, and over your wrists, as shown.

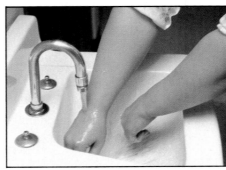

3 Now, you're ready to rinse your hands. To do this, place your hands under warm, running water. Point your fingertips downward to prevent bacteria from running onto your forearms and becoming a possible source of infection. Make sure you don't touch the sides of the sink. If you do, wash your hands again.

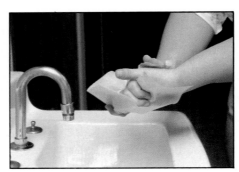

4 Now, dry your hands with a paper towel, as the nurse is doing in this photo. Discard the paper towel.

Suppose your sink doesn't have foot or knee controls for the water. In this case, turn off the faucets with the paper towel before discarding it.

Cleaning, disinfecting, and sterilizing

Hand washing: Some helpful tips

On page 79, we showed you how to wash your hands properly. Now, let's review some basic hand-washing guidelines:

When to use soap:
- before coming on duty
- before and after direct or indirect patient contact
- before and after performing any body functions, such as blowing your nose or going to the toilet
- before preparing or serving food and medications
- after completing your shift.

When to use antiseptic:
- after direct or indirect contact with a patient's excreta, secreta, or blood
- before and after catheter and I.V. insertions
- before and after dressing changes
- before and after caring for patients with suspected infection, in high-risk areas, or in isolation.

Additional guidelines:
Here are some more hand-washing tips:
- Clean under your fingernails with an orange stick or brush before and after working in high-risk areas.
- Avoid hand cream while working. It may interfere with the antiseptic solution.
- Always wash your hands before putting on clean or sterile gloves and after removing them. Torn gloves may allow your hands to become contaminated, or allow your hands to contaminate your patient.

How to properly care for a liquid soap dispenser

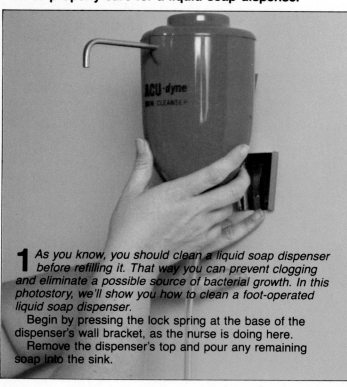

1 *As you know, you should clean a liquid soap dispenser before refilling it. That way you can prevent clogging and eliminate a possible source of bacterial growth. In this photostory, we'll show you how to clean a foot-operated liquid soap dispenser.*

Begin by pressing the lock spring at the base of the dispenser's wall bracket, as the nurse is doing here.

Remove the dispenser's top and pour any remaining soap into the sink.

2 Now, check the nozzle opening for clogging. If you see any dry soap residue, clean the opening with a paper clip or applicator stick, as shown.

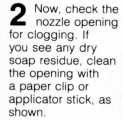
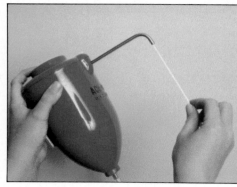

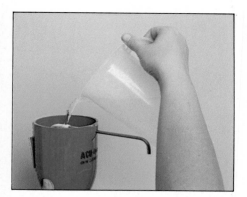

3 Fill the dispenser with warm water. Now, step on the pedal several times. Doing so will flush water through the dispenser.

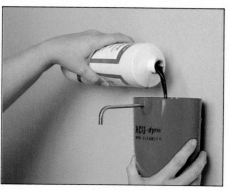

4 Pour remaining water into the sink. Then, reposition the dispenser on the wall bracket.

Next, pour liquid soap into the dispenser until the soap is about ¾" (1.9 cm) from the top of the dispenser.

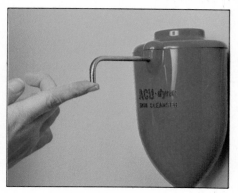

5 To deliver soap to the nozzle, step down on the foot pedal as you place your finger over the nozzle opening. Then, release pressure on the foot pedal.

Repeat this procedure several times until soap comes out of the nozzle.

Note: When used infrequently, some liquid soaps may discolor.

Nurses' guide to disinfectants

Disinfectants vary in strength and effectiveness against specific pathogens. Before choosing a disinfectant, consider the article to be disinfected and how it's used; what pathogens may be present; and the required level of disinfection. For example, articles that are invasive, or that enter sterile areas of the body, require a high level of disinfection or sterilization.

In addition, remember these guidelines:
- Disassemble article, if possible, before cleaning and disinfecting.
- If you're using a detergent/disinfectant compound solution, clean the article before disinfection.

- Make a fresh disinfectant solution, whenever possible, according to the manufacturer's directions. Always mark the bottle with the time and date prepared, your initials, and the manufacturer's recommended expiration date.
- Never add fresh disinfectant solution to an already prepared solution.
- Always store the disinfectant solution in the proper container and storage area, according to manufacturer's recommendations.

For more information on specific types of disinfectants, read the chart that follows.

Agent	Purpose	Nursing considerations
Isopropyl alcohol (70 to 90%)	• Bactericidal • Effective against gram-positive and gram-negative organisms, and *Mycobacterium tuberculosis*. Ineffective against spores.	• To avoid skin irritation, wear gloves when using. • Don't immerse rubber or plastic articles. • Because alcohol evaporates quickly, use disinfected object immediately. Remember, agent loses effectiveness when evaporated.
Chlorine (modified Dakin's solution)	• Bactericidal • Effective against gram-negative organisms, *Mycobacterium tuberculosis*, spores, hepatitis virus, and some gram-positive organisms. • Used for patient-care equipment, such as bedpans, urinals, and thermometers; as well as for special general housekeeping chores. Also used in dialysis areas.	• To avoid skin irritation, wear gloves when using. Also, don't use on items having close contact with patient's mucous membranes. • Avoid using on metal articles to prevent discoloration and corrosion (in some cases). • Prepare fresh solution each time and use it immediately. Discard what remains.
Formaldehyde (in alcohol 70%)	• Bactericidal • Effective against gram-positive and gram-negative organisms, *Mycobacterium tuberculosis*, spores, and hepatitis virus.	• To avoid skin irritation, wear gloves when using. Also, don't use on items that have close contact with the patient's mucous membranes. • Releases a pungent odor; use in a ventilated area.
Formalin (40% formaldehyde in water)	• Bactericidal • Effective against gram-positive and gram-negative organisms, and *Mycobacterium tuberculosis*. Less effective against spores.	• Rinse article after disinfecting. • Releases a pungent odor that may irritate eyes, nose, and throat. Always use in well-ventilated room.
Glutaraldehyde Cidex 7™ Cidex™	• Bactericidal • Effective against gram-positive and gram-negative organisms, *Mycobacterium tuberculosis*, viruses and bacterial spores. • Used to disinfect respiratory therapy equipment, lensed instruments, polyethylene tubing, and dialysis equipment.	• To avoid skin irritation, wear gloves when using. • Store in a cool place. • Use in a well-ventilated room. • Activate before using. When activated, agent changes color. • Read manufacturer's instructions carefully. • Immerse article in agent (2% alkaline) for about 10 hours to ensure effectiveness against bacterial spores.
Iodophor Pharmadine®	• Bactericidal • Effective against gram-positive and gram-negative organisms, and some viruses. Less effective against *Mycobacterium tuberculosis*. • Use for patient-care equipment, such as bedpans and urinals; as well as for general housekeeping.	• Avoid using on metal articles, to prevent discoloration and corrosion (in some cases). • In high concentrations, agent may temporarily stain equipment.
Phenol O-Syl® Tergisyl®	• Bactericidal • Effective against gram-positive and gram-negative organisms, some viruses, and *Mycobacterium tuberculosis*. Less effective against spores. • Used for patient-care equipment, such as bedpans, and urinals, as well as for general housekeeping.	• To avoid skin irritation, wear gloves when using. Don't use on articles that have close contact with the patient's mucous membranes. • Reactivates when exposed to moisture.
QUATS (quaternary ammonium compounds) Detergicide Consan Instrument Germicide	• Bactericidal • Effective against gram-positive organisms. Less effective against gram-negative organisms, and ineffective against *Mycobacterium tuberculosis* and spores. • Used for patient-care equipment, such as bedpans and urinals, as well as for general housekeeping.	• Avoid using with soap. Soap reduces agent's effectiveness. • Do not use for antisepsis. • Pour directly on item to be cleaned. Cleaning cloths will absorb agent.

Cleaning, disinfecting, and sterilizing

Cleaning a soiled article: Speculum

1 *The doctor's just finished performing a pelvic exam on your patient. In your hospital cleaning a soiled article, such as a speculum, is a nursing responsibility. Here's how to proceed:*

First, rinse the speculum with cool water and bring it to the dirty utility room. Then, make sure you have the following equipment available: disposable gloves, brush with stiff bristles, basin, detergent for cleaning the speculum (such as Sklar-Kleen®), antiseptic cleaning agent for hand washing, and paper towels.

Slip the gloves onto your hands.

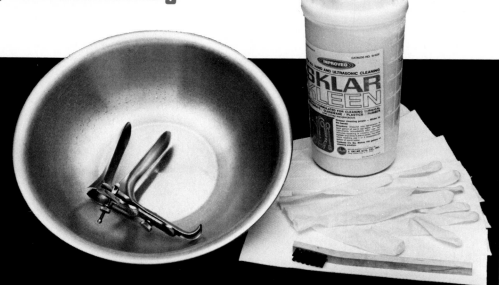

2 Put the measured detergent into the basin, following manufacturer's instructions. Add the proper amount of water.

Now, place the speculum in the basin. To make cleaning easier, let it soak for a few minutes.

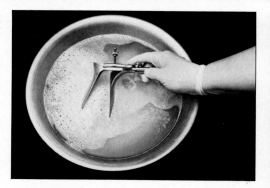

3 Then, scrub the speculum with a paper towel, loosening accumulated secretions.

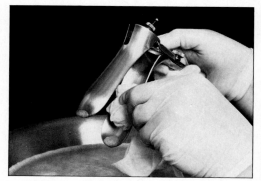

4 If any remain, use the bristled brush to remove them. But, be careful not to splash the water. Doing so may spread contaminated droplets.

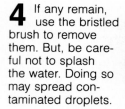

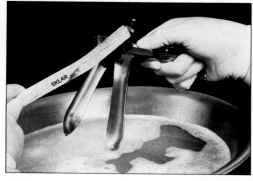

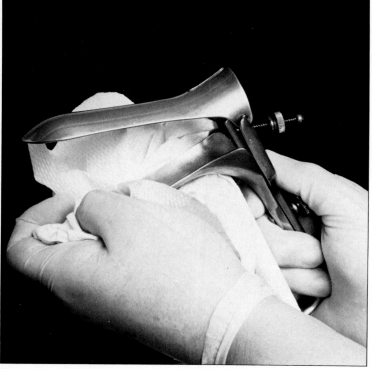

5 Next, rinse the speculum under hot water to remove loosened secretions. The heat of the water also will help to dry the speculum.

Now, using a clean paper towel, dry the speculum. Discard the towel in the covered wastebasket.

Is the speculum disposable? If so, rinse it with water before discarding it. This eliminates a source of bacterial growth.

Depending on hospital policy, you may want to clean the basin and bristled brush before bringing the speculum to the utility room to wrap. If this is the case, place the speculum on a clean paper towel. Then, cover the speculum with another clean paper towel.

Then, remove your gloves and discard them in the covered wastebasket. Wash your hands with cleaning antiseptic.

Learning about sterilization methods

Has it been a while since you reviewed sterilization methods? No matter how your hospital sterilizes equipment, you should be familiar with all available methods.

As you know, the best sterilization method for any article is one that reliably destroys all microorganisms or spores without damaging the article.

To learn about the advantages and disadvantages of different sterilization methods, study the following chart.

Type	Advantages	Disadvantages
Heat Saturated steam under pressure Sterilizes in approximately 15 minutes at 250° F. (121° C.).	• Can reach a temperature higher than boiling, because of pressure. • Destroys all forms of organisms by permeating the article with steam.	• Can't sterilize all articles; for example, heat-sensitive items such as syringes. • Pressure and heat intensity may dull sharp instruments.
Heat Boiling water Sterilizes in approximately 30 minutes at 212° F. (100° C.).	• Does not require special equipment. • Allows easy temperature control. • Available for home use.	• Does not destroy all viruses or any spores. • Not recommended for hospital use.
Heat Dry heat Sterilizes in approximately 1 hour at 320° F. (160° C.).	• Sterilizes articles damaged by moist heat; for example, syringes and sharp instruments. • Sterilizes powders, greases, and anhydrous oils.	• Before sterilization begins, preheat article to 320° F. (160° C.) for about 2 hours.
Chemical Gas (ethylene oxide) Sterilizes in approximately 5 hours at 70 to 140° F. (21° to 60° C.).	• Sterilizes articles damaged by moist and dry heat; for example, porous materials, delicate surgical instruments, and large pieces of equipment. • Destroys all microorganisms. • Does not require high temperature or pressure. • Does not corrode or damage article.	• Releases toxic fumes, requiring outside ventilation (not within hospital). • After sterilization, requires complete aeration of article, at least 24 hours in a room or 8 to 12 hours in an aeration cabinet, depending on the type of material. Some plastics may take longer. • If article's not sufficiently aerated, remaining chemical may irritate or burn skin.
Liquid Aqueous glutaraldehyde 2% Article must be completely immersed for 10 hours to sterilize.	• Sterilizes articles damaged by moist or dry heat, such as lenses and sharp instruments.	• After sterilization, article requires thorough rinsing with sterile water. • Irritates skin and mucous membranes. • Requires adequate room ventilation during sterilization.
Liquid Formaldehyde (Formalin); 37% aqueous solution formaldehyde Article must be completely immersed for 18 hours to kill resistant spores.	• Sterilizes dialysis machine of patient with hepatitis B.	• Releases a pungent odor. • Corrodes metal articles. • After sterilization, article requires thorough rinsing with sterile water. • Irritates skin and mucous membranes. • Requires adequate room ventilation during sterilization.

Cleaning, disinfecting, and sterilizing

Cleaning a soiled article: Some reminders

You know how important it is to properly clean a soiled article. Cleaning removes contaminants, such as a patient's excretions, which may interfere with disinfection and sterilization procedures.

When cleaning an article, use detergent rather than soap. Why? Detergent attacks bacteria with minimal scrubbing and leaves no residue to interfere with the disinfectant's effectiveness. If the article's heavily soiled, use a scrub brush with detergent.

Of course, sometimes you may not have time to properly clean a soiled article. In this case, rinse the article and let it soak in disinfectant. When you have more time, complete the cleaning procedure.

Remember: Never leave a soiled article on a table. This provides a reservoir for bacteria.

Preparing a lightweight article for sterilization: A small ring forceps

1 *Let's assume you've just cleaned a small ring forceps. If wrapping an instrument for sterilization is a nursing responsibility in your hospital, follow these steps:*

First, you'll need a paper-plastic pouch, such as the Ameri-Wrap® self-sealing package for gas and steam sterilization. This pouch has steam-autoclaving and gas-sterilization chemical indicator strips impregnated on the wrapper. By changing color during the sterilization process, each strip monitors the appropriate sterilization time, temperature, and saturation level.

Note: If this sterilization package is unavailable, follow your hospital's wrapping policy.

Label the paper side of the package with the name of the article and your initials. Following your hospital's policy, check the forcep's shelf life after sterilization. Mark the expiration date on the pouch. If your hospital uses lot numbers, be sure to note the correct area number on the package.

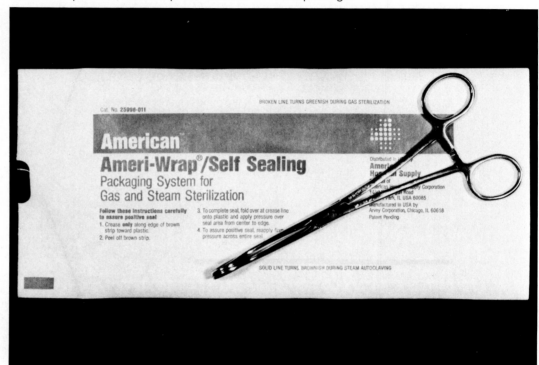

2 Place the opened forceps into the pouch. Check that the forceps is completely opened to ensure thorough sterilization.

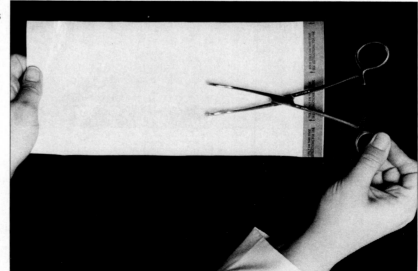

3 Moving along the edge of the brown strip, fold the paper wrap down over the plastic, as shown. Then, unfold the wrapper edge.

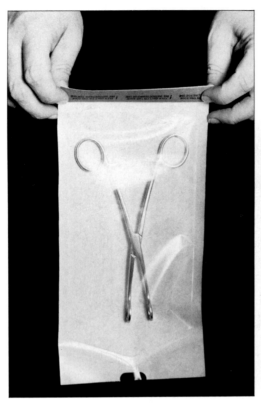

5 Fold over the package at the creased line. Secure the seal by applying even fingertip pressure from the seal's center to the edges, as shown.

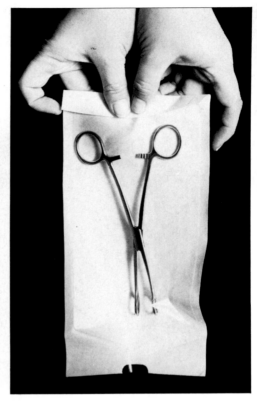

4 Now, peel off the brown strip, as the nurse is doing in this photo.

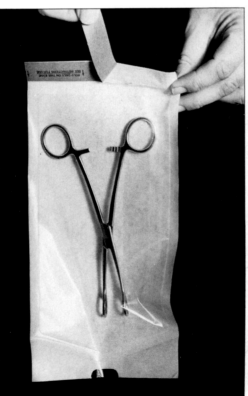

6 To ensure a firm seal, reapply even fingertip pressure across the entire seal.
Finally, bring the properly prepared forceps to central supply service for sterilization. Or, follow your hospital's policy.

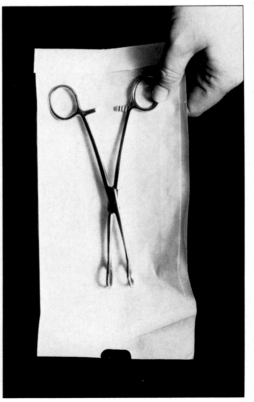

Cleaning, disinfecting, and sterilizing

Preparing an article for sterilization: Double wrapping method

1 *Imagine this situation: 25-year-old Bernard Olsen, a patient with second-degree burns, has been transferred from the ICU to your floor. Because he's in protective isolation, all his linens must be sterilized. If your hospital doesn't use prepackaged sterile burn packs, you'll need to wrap clean linens from the laundry for sterilization. In this photostory, the nurse will be double wrapping Mr. Olsen's gown. Here's how:*

First, bring the gown to the utility room or wrapping area, following your hospital's policy.

Then, assemble the necessary equipment: sterilization wrap, steam indicator strip, and autoclave tape. The nurse in this photostory will be using Dextex® II sterilization wrap, a Castle Tec-Test steam sterilization integrator and a felt-tipped pen.

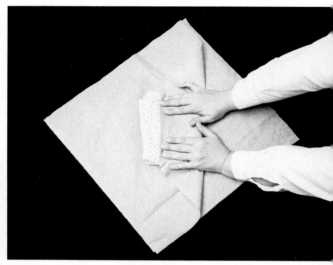

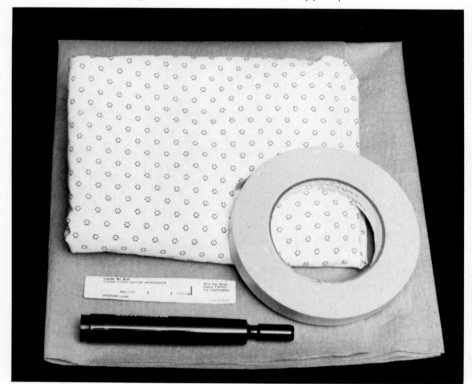

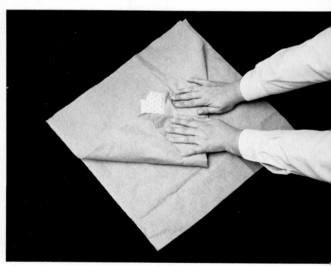

2 Holding the two wrappers together, position them diagonally on a table.

Center the patient gown on the top wrapper. Place the steam sterilization integrator on top of the patient gown, as the nurse is doing here.

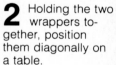

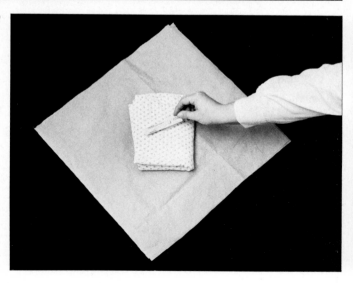

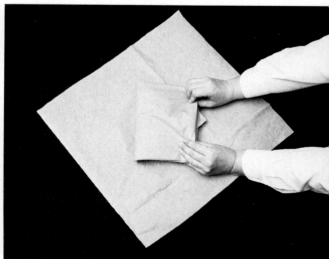

3 Next, fold the top wrapper's corner closest to you over the patient gown, as shown.
Fanfold the corner to make a tab.

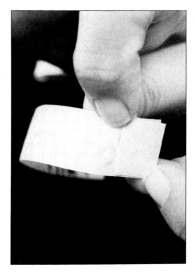

6 Next, cut a piece of autoclave tape long enough to secure the top flap and wrap it 2″ to 3″ (5.1 to 7.6 cm) around the back.
Fold the first ½″ (1.3 cm) of tape back on itself, forming a tab.

4 Fold the left corner over the patient gown. Then, fold the right corner over.
Note: In some hospitals, all three corners are fanfolded.

5 Now, fold down the remaining corner, as the nurse is doing here. Tuck the end under the folded wrapper.
Repeat the entire procedure with the outside wrapper.

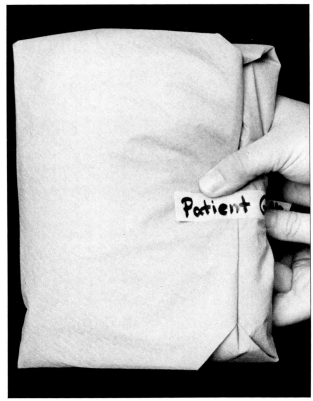

7 Holding the tape tab on the top flap, wrap the tape around the bottom of the wrapper, as shown here.
Now, following your hospital's policy, note the last date the gown can be used safely, and mark the expiration date, the article's name, and your initials on the wrapper. If your hospital uses lot numbers, also be sure to mark the correct area number on the wrapper.
Take the wrapped article to the floor sterilizer or to central supply service, following hospital policy.

Wrapping an article for sterilization: Some guidelines

Is wrapping an article for sterilization a nursing responsibility in your hospital? If so, here are some reminders:
• Always use freshly laundered muslin to wrap an article. Worn or soiled muslin may interfere with the sterilization process.
• Paper-plastic pouches or paper also are acceptable wrap.
• Use autoclave tape to seal the wrapped article. Avoid using other closures, such as rubber bands, pins, or paper clips, which increase the possibility of contamination.
• When wrapping basin sets, place absorbent towels between each basin to allow full steam permeation.
• Do not mix basins, trays, and metal articles with linen packs. Doing so interferes with the linen pack's sterilization.
• Before wrapping surgical instruments, place them in a tray with a wire-mesh bottom. Make sure all instruments are open, unlocked, or disassembled.

MINI-ASSESSMENT

Learning when to replace sterile supplies

Do you know why it's important to routinely check storage supply areas on your floor? Because using outdated or damaged sterile supplies may be an infection source. Always return sterile supplies to central supply service to obtain replacements when you see:
• past-due expiration dates on package
• open or torn wrappers
• broken seals
• cracked bottles.
In addition, you'll want to observe the following important measures:
• rotate duplicate articles by placing the most recently produced article behind the older one.
• keep stock cabinets closed, and carts or shelves covered, when not in use.
Remember: You can extend the shelf life of infrequently used supplies 6 to 18 months by using a dustcover. Always use dustcovers in high-risk areas; for example, in a burn unit or operating room.

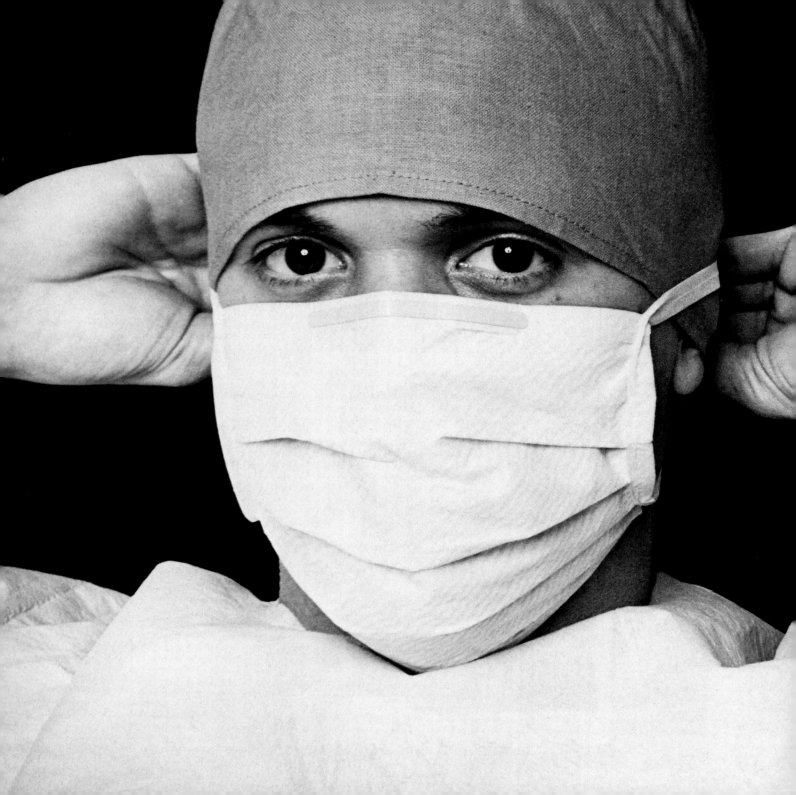

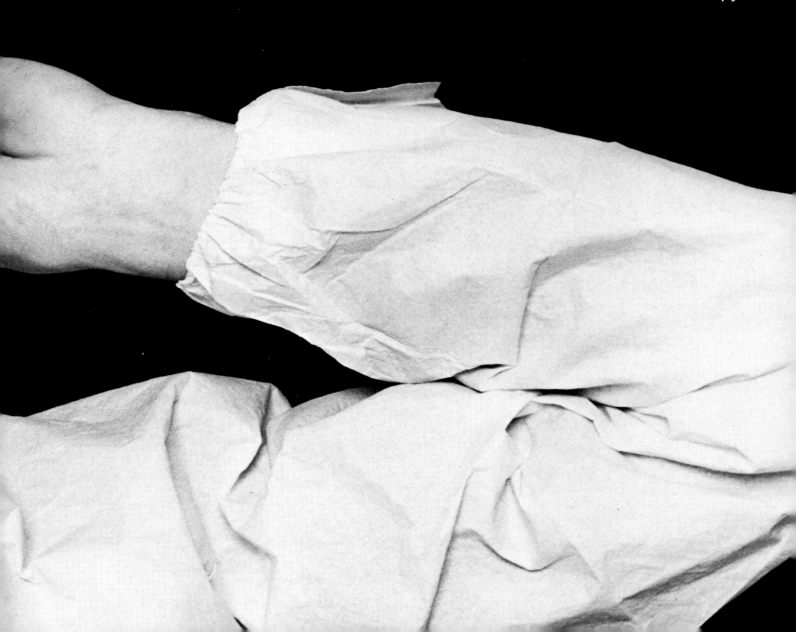

Limiting Infection

Isolation procedures

Antibiotic therapy

Isolation procedures

How familiar are you with isolation procedures? For example, do you know how to put on isolation gloves, mask and gown? Or, how to remove them when they're contaminated? Do you know how to set up an isolation room? Or how to terminally disinfect an isolation room when your patient's discharged?

What about caring for the patient? Do you know how you can make his stay in isolation more pleasant? Or, how to help his family cope with the situation?

In this section, we'll answer these questions and provide additional information that'll help you do your job better. Study the following pages carefully.

Understanding isolation

As you probably know, isolation precautions help prevent the spread of infection. But do you know how?

The basic principle of isolation is simple. Before an infection can spread, an agent, mode of transmission, and a susceptible host must exist. Isolation precautions break the transmission link in the chain of infection.

In many hospitals, you'll take the necessary isolation precautions as soon as a communicable situation is suspected, or diagnosed. Then, depending on your hospital's policy, you may need to obtain a doctor's order.

Of course, making the decision to place a patient in isolation isn't easy. Why? Because placing a patient in isolation is time-consuming to all hospital personnel. It also increases your patient's hospitalization costs.

Isolation precautions mean extra supplies. And, in some cases, a longer hospital stay. Doctors, nurses, aides, and housekeeping staff members will need extra time to put on and remove the appropriate isolation garb and obtain, remove and transport the necessary equipment. In some cases, the patient may be placed in a private room, which deprives him of companionship and social interaction.

But, always consider the advantages of isolation. By isolating a patient with a communicable condition or disease you'll reduce the spread of infection and may prevent additional health risks for all involved.

Nurses' guide to isolation precautions

Your patient has an infectious disease and needs to be placed in isolation. How do you know which type of isolation is best suited to his condition? That depends on your hospital. However, the Center for Disease Control (CDC) in Atlanta has established guidelines for the five degrees (levels) of isolation: strict, respiratory, enteric, protective, and wound and skin.

In designating these guidelines, the CDC has attempted to weigh the disadvantages of isolation with the potential danger of communicable conditions. Of course, you may need to modify these guidelines in some situations, such as when:
• a patient needs constant care; for example, a critical patient in the isolation room of an intensive care unit.
• an emergency situation develops while a patient's in isolation; for example, a cardiac arrest.

But, you'll need to take isolation precautions when your patient's condition has the potential to be infectious to others; for example, if a patient with a bladder infection and an indwelling catheter is in a room with a patient with an indwelling catheter but no bladder infection.

When you need to modify established isolation procedures, keep in mind that your objective is to minimize the risk of spreading infection to other patients and other personnel.

Take a look at the chart which follows. It describes the five isolation levels as designated by the CDC, and some nursing considerations for each level. But remember, whenever you care for a patient in isolation, always follow your hospital's policy.

Strict isolation

Purpose
• Prevents transmission of highly communicable diseases spread by direct contact, and airborne microorganisms.

Recommended for patients with *Staphylococcus aureus* and group A *streptococcus* infections on wounds, burns, and skin when dressing is not used or does not adequately absorb purulent drainage; or when extensive dermatitis exists.

Disease requiring isolation
• Inhalation anthrax
• Diphtheria
• Neonatal vesicular disease (herpes simplex)
• Rabies
• Congenital rubella syndrome
• Disseminated herpes zoster or herpes zoster when unable to cover sores with dressings
• Pneumonia with *Staphylococcus aureus* or group A *streptococcus*
• Chicken pox
• Lassa fever
• Marburg virus disease
• Smallpox
• Pneumonic plague

Nursing considerations
• Place patient in a private room with slight negative air pressure and an anteroom (if possible). Keep door closed at all times. If necessary put an exhaust fan in the window to help improve air circulation and pressure.
• Employees and visitors entering isolation room must wear gown, mask, and gloves.
• Wash hands before entering and after leaving room, and during patient care.
• Clean and double bag contaminated articles from room before sending them to central supply department for disinfection or sterilization. Also, double bag patient's clothes and send home with family. Be sure to include washing instructions.
• Make sure all susceptible employees are vaccinated or immune before caring for a patient with rubella or diphtheria.
• Place all linen in a water-soluble bag.
• Don't transport patient from his room unless necessary.
• Use disposable needles and syringes, if possible. Discard used needles in puncture-resistant container.
• Pin an impervious plastic bag to the patient's bedside for tissue disposal.
• Place all soiled dressings, tissues, and other disposable articles in a wastebasket lined with an impervious plastic bag. As soon as possible, remove bag from room, using the double-bag technique. Discard according to hospital policy.
• Carefully label all containers and specimen bottles CONTAMINATED or ISOLATION to alert other employees to possible contamination.
• Keep patient's chart *outside* of the isolation room.

Respiratory isolation

Purpose
• Prevents transmission of communicable diseases spread by direct or indirect contact, or airborne microorganisms spread by droplets exhaled, coughed or sneezed into the air.

Disease requiring isolation
• Rubeola (measles)
• Meningococcal meningitis
• Meningococcemia
• Mumps
• Pertussis (whooping cough)
• Rubella (German measles)
• Active pulmonary tuberculosis, including the respiratory tract. Suspected or confirmed sputum-positive smear.

Nursing considerations
• If possible, place patient in a private room with a slight negative pressure and an anteroom. If necessary, two patients with identical infections may share a room. Keep door closed at all times. If necessary, put an exhaust fan in the window to help improve air circulation and pressure.
• Employees and visitors entering isolation room must wear a mask.
• Wash hands before entering, and after leaving room, and during patient care.
• Instruct patient to use a tissue to cover his mouth and nose when coughing or sneezing.
• Pin an impervious plastic bag to the patient's bedside for tissue disposal.
• Place all soiled dressings and tissues in a wastebasket lined with an impervious plastic bag and discard following hospital policy.
• If patient has pulmonary tuberculosis, place sputum specimen in an impervious specimen container with a secure lid. Label specimen appropriately.
• Advise susceptible pregnant employees to avoid work in the newborn infant nursery, pediatric unit, emergency department, and outpatient clinic. Doing so prevents possible exposure to rubella.
• Check that all susceptible personnel are vaccinated and given recommended booster inoculations before caring for a patient with mumps, measles, or German measles.
• If patient must be transported, notify his destination area for necessary isolation precautions. Also, check to make sure the patient is wearing a mask.
• Clean and wrap reusable equipment for inhalation therapy. Send articles to the central supply department for proper disinfection and reprocessing, or discard according to hospital policy.

Protective isolation

Purpose
• Prevents contact between potentially infectious organisms and patients who run a high risk of contracting an infection because of certain diseases, therapeutic regimens, or other conditions.

Disease requiring isolation
• Agranulocytosis
• Extensive, noninfected burns (in certain patients)
• Dermatitis, noninfected vesicular, bullous, or eczematous disease (when severe and extensive)
• In some case, lymphomas and leukemia, specifically in late stages of Hodgkin's disease or acute leukemia; low white blood count

Nursing considerations
• Isolate patient only as ordered.
• Place patient in a private room with positive air pressure and an anteroom. Keep door closed at all times.
• Disinfect the impervious plastic covering mattress and pillow covers immediately before patient's arrival in isolation room.
• Use only sterile linen.
• Screen employees and visitors entering patient's room for fever blisters, infections, or colds. If present, do not allow them to enter room. Try to limit individuals entering room.
• Employees and visitors entering isolation room must wear a sterile gown, mask and gloves (for direct patient contact). Use caps and shoe covers, following hospital policy. Some hospitals may require sterile isolation garb.
• If possible, avoid performing invasive procedures that increase risk of infections; for example, catheterization.
• Don't transport patient from room, unless necessary.
• If invasive procedures must be performed, maintain *strict* aseptic technique at all times.
• Any article brought into patient's room must be sterile or highly disinfected.

Isolation procedures

Nurses' guide to isolation precautions continued

Enteric precautions

Purpose
• Prevents transmission of communicable disease spread by direct or indirect contact with infected feces, and in some cases, heavily contaminated articles, such as bedpans.

Disease requiring isolation
• Cholera
• Diarrhea, and acute illness caused by a suspected infection.
• Enterocolitis caused by staphylococci
• Gastroenteritis caused by enteropathogenic or enterotoxic *Escherichia coli. Salmonella* species including *Salmonella typhi* (typhoid fever), *Shigella* species, or *Yersinia enterocolitica*
• Viral hepatitis, type A, type B, or type non-A/non-B

Nursing considerations
• Isolate newborn infants who have clinical or suspected gastroenteritis, or suspected infectious diarrhea.
• If patient's continent and well-adjusted, allow him to share toilet facilities with other patients, after proper instructions. Follow your hospital's policy.
• Place confused adult patients, as well as pediatric patients with fecal incontinence, in private rooms.
• Make sure employees and visitors wear gown and gloves if they have direct contact with patient, or with article contaminated with patient's feces.
• Wash hands before entering and after leaving isolation area and during patient care.
• Instruct patient to wash hands thoroughly, especially after using the toilet.
• Clean any article contaminated with patient's urine or feces. Then, disinfect article with a germicide.
• When caring for a patient with viral hepatitis, use disposable needles and syringes, if possible. Discard used needles into puncture-resistant container. Never bend or break used needle. If using reusable needles or syringes, rinse needle under cold water after using. Place in an impervious container. Double bag the needle and syringe, label the bag HEPATITIS, and send to the central supply department.
• Pin an impervious plastic bag at the patient's bedside for tissue disposal.
• Place all soiled dressings, tissues, and other soiled disposable articles in a wastebasket lined with an impervious plastic bag. As soon as possible, remove and discard it, following hospital policy.
• If patient uses a bedpan or urinal, empty contents directly into toilet. Then, clean bedpan or urinal and return it to the patient's bedside. When patient's discharged, wrap the bedpan or urinal in an impervious plastic bag, close it securely, and label it CONTAMINATED or ISOLATION. Send to the central supply department.
• Place specimen in sterile container with secure lid. Double bag container, and label it CONTAMINATED or ISOLATION. Wipe outside of container with a disinfectant. Send to the lab. If patient has viral hepatitis, clearly label HEPATITIS on blood specimen container.
• Double bag removable instruments and equipment after cleaning, proper disinfection, and reprocessing, and send them to the central supply department for sterilization or disinfection. Use a germicide to wipe instruments and equipment that can't be removed.

Wound and skin precautions

Purpose
• Prevents transmission of infection between patients and employees by restricting direct contact with infected wounds, burns, and articles contaminated with infected wound drainage.

Disease requiring isolation
• Wound and skin infections other than those infected with *Staphylococcus aureus* or Group A *streptococcus* when not covered by dressing.
• Gas gangrene (from *Clostridium perfringens*)
• Localized herpes zoster
• Extrapulmonary melioidosis with draining sinuses
• Bubonic plague
• Puerperal sepsis with Group A *streptococcus* and vaginal discharge

Nursing considerations
• Place patient in a private room, if possible.
• Employees must wear gowns, sterile gloves, and mask when having direct contact with patient's infected area.
• Wash hands before entering and after leaving isolation room; also, before and after patient care.
• After removing soiled dressing, remove gloves, wash your hands, and put on clean, sterile gloves. Use sterile surgical instruments to pick up and apply clean dressings.
• Place soiled dressings in an impervious plastic bag. Close bag securely, double bag, and discard, following hospital policy.
• Double bag patient's clothing and send home with family. Be sure to include washing instructions.
• Instruct visitors to avoid touching the patient's dressings, linens, or infected skin.
• Before transporting patient, cover infected area with a fresh dressing. For additional protection, place a sterile towel over the dressing. Also, be sure to notify destination area for necessary isolation precautions.

Learning about an anteroom

The anteroom plays an important part in controlling infection. Located between an isolation room and the hallway, the anteroom serves as an infection barrier. Why? Consider these three reasons. When the door to the isolation room's open, the anteroom helps reduce the spread of airborne infectious microorganisms into the hallway. Why? Because air pressure in the hall and anteroom is greater than in the isolation room (reverse is true in protective isolation). And anyone entering or leaving the isolation room must use the anteroom's cleaning and disinfecting facilities, minimizing the spread of infection through direct or indirect contact. Finally, the anteroom provides a covered storage space for isolation supplies, to prevent contamination.

What's in an anteroom? Usually you'll find hand-washing facilities and a storage area for necessary isolation supplies. In most hospitals, keeping the anteroom stocked with isolation supplies is a nursing responsibility.

Wondering what supplies you need? Make sure you have enough isolation masks, gloves (sterile and nonsterile), caps, and gowns for both you and your patient's visitors. You'll also need the appropriate isolation sign for the door and supplies for removing contaminated articles, such as linen, trash, and other equipment. These necessary supplies include: linen hampers, water-soluble linen bags, plastic trash bags, clear plastic bags, isolation stickers, germicidal agent, and emesis basins.

Is your patient in protective isolation? If so, you'll need sterile supplies as well, including sheets, pillowcases, patient gowns, isolation garb, towels, and washcloths.

Of course, not all hospitals require the same anteroom supplies. Follow your hospital's policy. And remember, not every isolation room has an anteroom. An isolation cart equipped with hand-washing liquids that don't require water and supply space may serve as an anteroom.

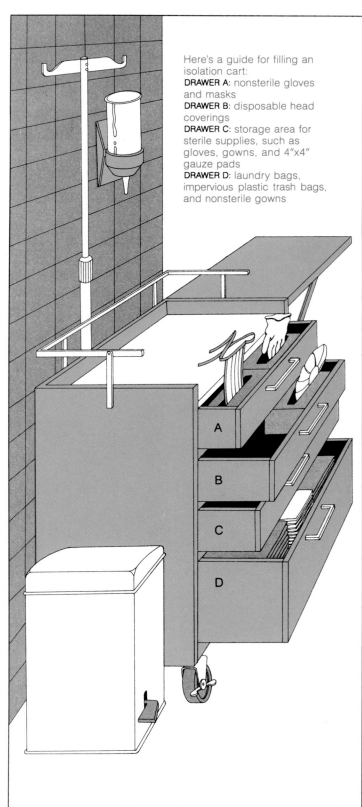

Here's a guide for filling an isolation cart:
DRAWER A: nonsterile gloves and masks
DRAWER B: disposable head coverings
DRAWER C: storage area for sterile supplies, such as gloves, gowns, and 4"x4" gauze pads
DRAWER D: laundry bags, impervious plastic trash bags, and nonsterile gowns

Using an isolation cart

Do you work in a hospital where an isolation cart is used instead of an anteroom? If so, you may use an isolation cart like the one shown at left.

As you know, an isolation cart is *always* kept outside of the isolation room. The cart may be a covered utility table with wheels, or it may be specially designed for isolation purposes. The isolation cart should include a work area (such as a pull-out shelf); drawers or a cabinet for isolation supplies; and possibly a pole to hang coats or jackets. Alongside the cart should be a covered trash receptacle.

The isolation cart usually contains the same supplies as the anteroom. But, one major difference exists between the anteroom and isolation cart: hand-washing facilities.

Because the cart has no sink or running water, you'll use a wall-mounted dispenser with a skin-cleaning agent that does not require rinsing with water.

To use the wall-mounted dispenser, apply enough cleaning agent to thoroughly clean your hands. For 30 to 60 seconds, continually massage and distribute the agent over both hands, covering your fingers and cuticles. When you're finished, dry your hands.

Note: If your patient's in any type of isolation except strict, you may wash your hands in the patient's bathroom, according to hospital policy.

Important: Some isolation carts store the skin-cleaning agent in a container with a pump.

You'll need to clean the isolation cart regularly, according to hospital policy. To do this, remove the supplies, put them on a clean, dry surface, and wipe all cart surfaces with a disinfectant. At the end of your shift, replace necessary items. Also, check expiration dates of the sterile supplies.

When your patient's discharged or transferred to another unit, clean and disinfect the isolation cart, discard leftover supplies, and return the cart to the storage area.

Isolation procedures

How to set up an isolation room

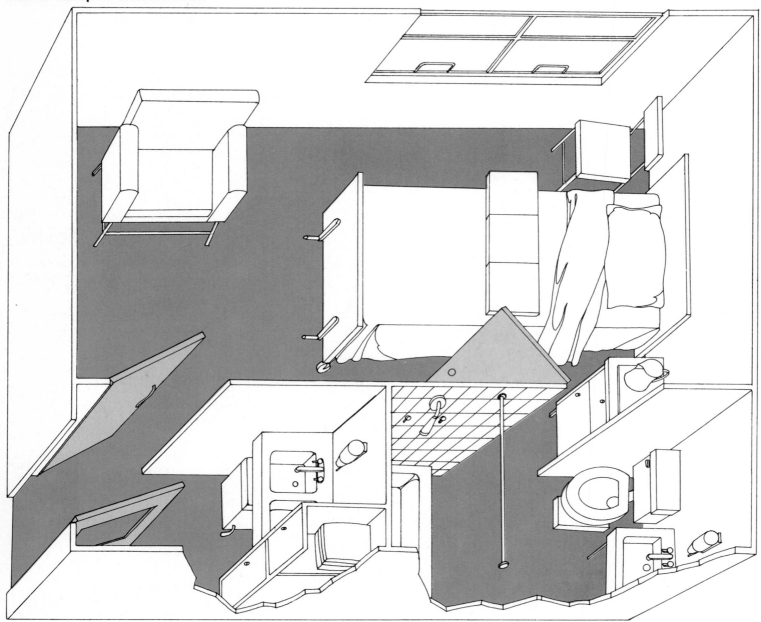

An isolation room serves a dual purpose in most hospitals. It may prevent the spread of an infectious disease. Or, it may protect a susceptible patient from becoming infected.

Any hospital room can be adapted for isolation purposes, even without proper facilities. Ideally, though, the room should have a bathroom with bathing facilities (as shown in this illustration). The bathroom eliminates the need for portable commodes. The isolation room door should open into the room and the room should be adequately ventilated.

In addition to the physical design, an isolation room requires special supplies. Before your patient arrives, you may be responsible for obtaining these supplies and properly preparing the room. If such is the case, remember these guidelines:

• Place the appropriate plasticized isolation card or identification card, and the appropriate visitor's card, on the room door.
• Cover the pillow with a plastic cover.
• Make sure the mattress is waterproof and plasticized. If it isn't, put on a plastic cover.
• On the bedside table, place a disposable pitcher and paper cups, tissues, and an individual thermometer in a holder.
• Pin an impervious plastic bag to the patient's bed for soiled tissue disposal.
• In the bathroom, place clean paper towels in the dispenser and fill the liquid soap dispenser with an antiseptic agent.
• When your patient arrives, place a covered linen stand and a wastebasket with an impervious plastic bag in the isolation room.

How to put on nonsterile isolation garb

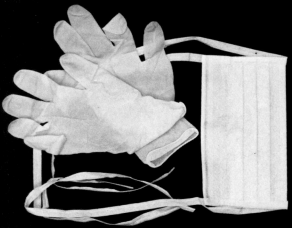 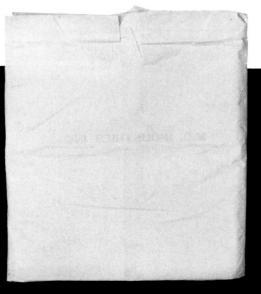

1 *In some hospitals, you may need to put on isolation garb before entering an isolation room. Here's the procedure:*
First, make sure your patient's anteroom or isolation cart has the following supplies (appropriate for the type of isolation he's in): gown (for example, an American Hospitex disposable gown, as shown here), gloves, and mask. You'll also need alcohol preps or antiseptic agent (such as Acu-Dyne), and paper towels.

2 Now, remove your watch. If your patient's room has no clock, carry the watch into the room on a clean paper towel, after you put on your isolation garb.
If your uniform has long sleeves, roll them up above your elbow to make sure your gown covers them completely. This protects your uniform from contamination.
Then, wash your hands thoroughly with an antiseptic cleaning agent and water. Dry them with a paper towel.

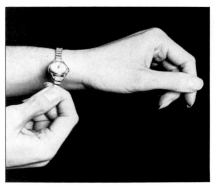

3 Next, unfold the gown with the opening facing you. Then, slip your arms through the gown's sleeves. Make sure the gown opening is in the back.
Adjust the cuffs so they fit comfortably on your wrists.

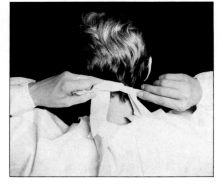

4 Position the gown around your neck. To help secure the gown, tie the neck strings as you would a shoelace.

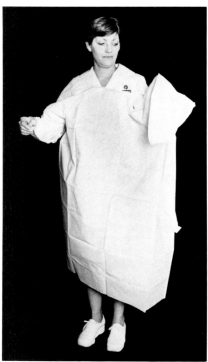 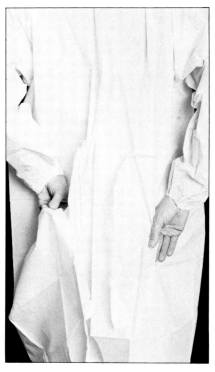

5 Now, overlap the back edges of the gown to protect your uniform. Then, tie the waist strings in the back, as the nurse is doing here. *Note:* If the waist strings are long enough, bring them around to the front and tie them together.

Isolation procedures

How to put on nonsterile isolation garb continued

6 Next, remove a face mask from the cabinet. With the metal strip facing outward, position the mask over your nose. Tie the mask's top strings just above the top of your ears, as shown here.

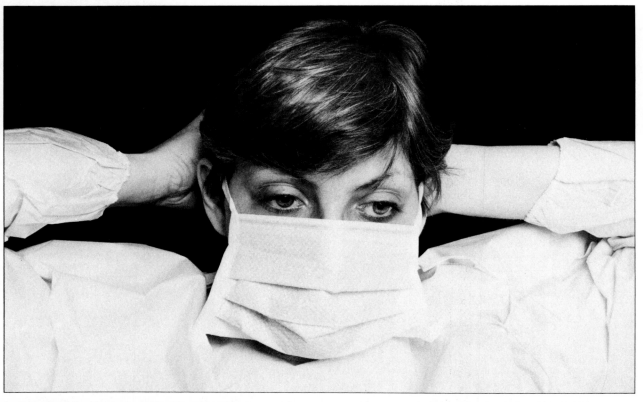

7 Pull down the lower part of the mask over your mouth and chin. Then, tie the bottom strings around your neck.

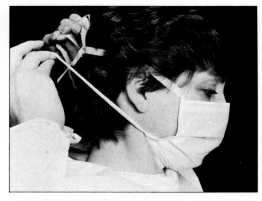

8 Press the metal strip over your nose so the mask fits comfortably and snugly.

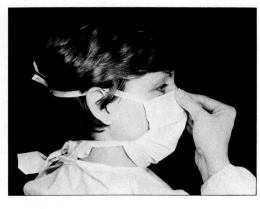

9 Now, slip the gloves onto your hands, making sure they fit snugly over the gown's cuffs.

☞ *Nursing tip:* Take an extra pair of gloves into the isolation room. By doing this, you can change your gloves immediately if they tear or become soiled. Place the extra pair on a clean paper towel, away from your patient.

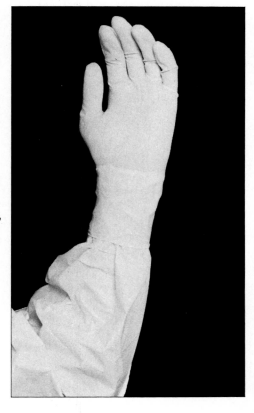

How to put on sterile gloves

1 *Before performing a procedure requiring aseptic technique, you'll need to put on sterile gloves. Here's how:*
First, remove all your jewelry. But, if you're wearing a plain wedding ring, you may keep it on. Then, wash your hands thoroughly and dry them with a paper towel.

Open the package containing the sterile gloves (see inset). Carefully open the inner wrapper, maintaining aseptic technique. Be very careful not to contaminate the gloves by touching them.
Now, grasp the folded edge of the right glove's cuff with your left hand, as shown in this photo.

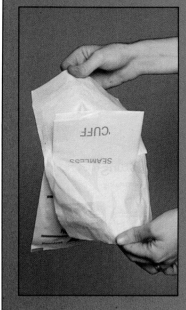
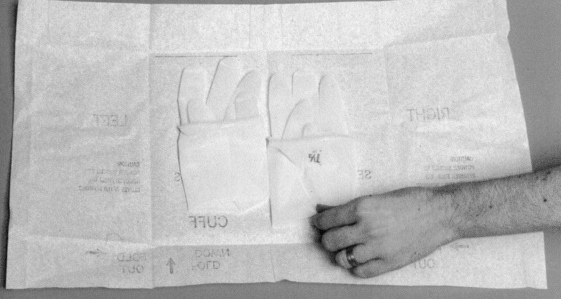

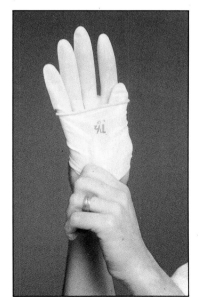

2 Slip your right hand inside the glove. To avoid contamination, be sure your left fingers touch only the inside of the glove. If the glove becomes contaminated, discard it and obtain a new one.

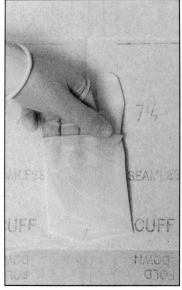

3 Next, slip the fingers of your gloved hand *under* the cuff of the left glove, as the nurse is doing here.

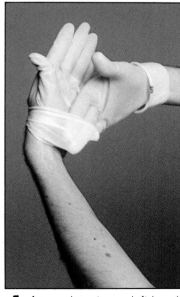

4 As you insert your left hand into the glove, pull the glove on with your right hand. Avoid touching your skin with your gloved right hand.

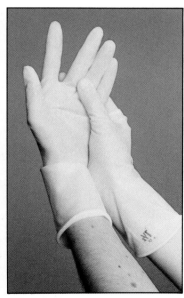

5 Finally, adjust both gloves so they fit properly. Make sure no gaps exist between your fingertips and the ends of the gloves. Inspect your gloves for nicks or tears. If you see any, obtain a new pair of sterile gloves.

Isolation procedures

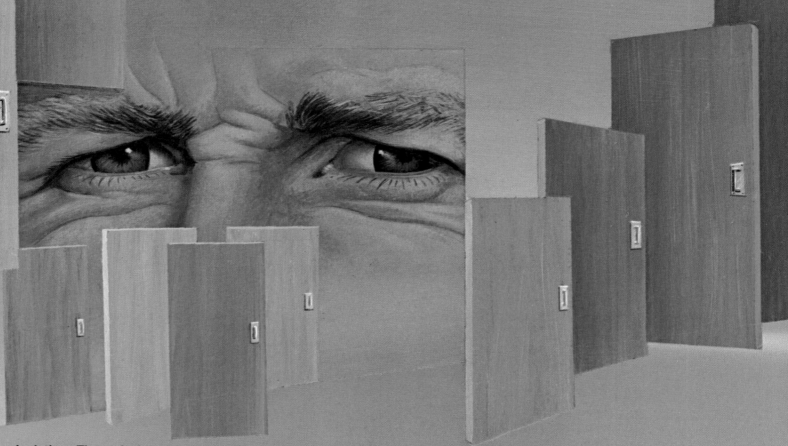

Isolation: Through the patient's eyes

A patient in isolation needs more than routine nursing care. Why? Because being in isolation can only intensify the loneliness of the hospital environment.

Consider the case of John Benson, a 29-year-old patient in strict isolation. He spends most of his hours alone in a room behind a closed door. Everyone who enters the room wears a barrier—mask, gown, and gloves—to protect themselves. Mr. Benson is scared and feels extremely depressed. But, with whom can he share his feelings?

Caring for the isolation patient's emotional needs is a large part of your nursing responsibility. How do you react to a patient in isolation? Do you find yourself avoiding him most of the day? Do you rush through his daily care because he requires more of your time than your other patients? Providing efficient care is important. But efficient care doesn't replace attention and emotional support.

When you first talk with Mr. Benson, he may act aggressive and uncooperative. Or, he may seem unusually quiet. These behaviors may be signs of his anxiety and apprehension.

To alleviate some of his fears, take time to explain why he's been placed in isolation. Find out what he knows about isolation and then attempt to clear up any misconceptions he may have. Encourage Mr. Benson to ask questions. Answer them as completely as possible. Try to understand the effect both his condition and isolation have on his emotions.

If your patient's a child or a teenager, he may be particularly upset. He may be in the hospital for the first time and probably misses his family. Try to take extra time reassuring him and explaining what isolation is. Attempt to anticipate his questions. Be sure to answer them clearly and completely.

Because much of any patient's social interaction will come from your visits, attempt to spend some time with him each day. As you perform your work, talk with him and touch his hand occasionally. Continually reassure him that isolation's only temporary. Try to gain his cooperation and trust. Emphasize how important his own personal hygiene is in preventing and controlling the spread of his infection.

To help improve your patient's morale, try incorporating some of these ideas into his care:
• Decorate the walls of his room with posters and paper decorations. Or, make him a calendar, which can be discarded later. Remember to mark off the days.
• Let him have some personal articles that can be easily disinfected; for example, a transistor radio. If your patient's a child, suggest his parents bring him an easily disinfected toy from home.
• Move the clock away from the patient's bed so he can't see it. His hours will be long enough without watching the minutes tick away.
• Encourage his family to visit. Recommend they bring your patient inexpensive gifts that will amuse him, such as magazines, paperback books, and puzzles.

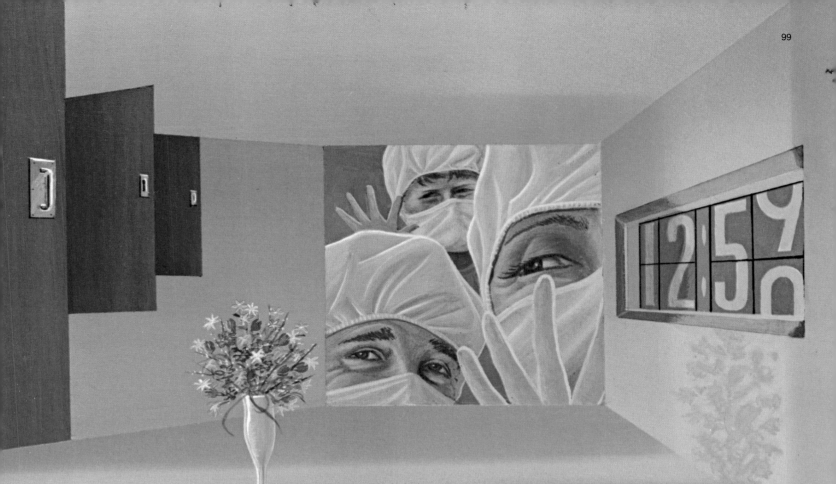

Teaching the family about isolation

After helping your patient adjust to isolation, talking to his family is your next responsibility. Doing so requires your time, empathy, patience, and energy. But, helping your patient's family understand isolation will also help your patient. Here are some guidelines to follow:

Explain to them in simple terms why the patient's been placed in isolation. If possible, let them know how long he'll be there.

Ask them how they feel about isolation. If they're uneasy about the patient's condition or his isolation environment, their attitudes may be picked up by the patient. Encourage them to share their feelings with you.

Try to find out what they know about isolation. For example, do they think isolation's only for seriously ill patients? Or, that they'll become infected if they enter the patient's room? Anticipate these concerns and clear up any misconceptions they may have.

Encourage the patient's family to visit as often as possible, according to hospital policy, provided they're in good health.

Make sure your patient's family understands that, although they will only have limited physical contact with the patient, they may bring him magazines, paperback books, and puzzles. Explain to them that any article that becomes contaminated may have to be discarded. Tell them to encourage friends and relatives to send the patient cards, and telephone (if he can receive calls). He'll probably be happy to receive the mail, and the phone calls will cheer him.

Explain that they'll have to take certain precautions to protect the patient and themselves from infection. Usually, these precautions will be performed in the anteroom (or near the isolation cart). Emphasize the importance of washing their hands before entering and after leaving the isolation room. Demonstrate how to put on and remove isolation garb properly. Then, ask them to put on and remove the garb.

Accompany them into the patient's room. Remind them not to sit on the patient's bed, touch the infected area, or use the patient's bathroom facilities.

Show them the proper receptacles for discarding isolation garb. Explain that these receptacles prevent cross-contamination and the spread of infection.

Teaching your patient infection control

Your patient in isolation can prevent his infection from spreading by observing these guidelines. Instruct him to:
• wash his hands with soap and water before eating, drinking, and after performing any body functions, such as using the toilet and blowing his nose.
• cover his nose and mouth with a tissue when he coughs or sneezes.
• discard used or soiled articles, such as tissues or hospital gowns, into the special containers in his room.
• bring as few personal belongings from home as possible.
• wear a hospital gown or pajamas instead of bringing bedclothes from home.
• use the call bell if he needs help. He should not leave his room without a doctor's or nurse's permission.

Isolation procedures

How to put on a sterile gown, mask, cap, and shoe covers

1 *Do you know the proper procedure for putting on a sterile gown, mask, cap and shoe covers? Follow these guidelines:*

First, obtain a sterile pack (we're using American Convertors Shield® Sterile Staff Pack) from your patient's anteroom or isolation cart. This pack includes a gown, mask, cap, and shoe covers. (In some hospitals these items are packaged individually.) You'll also need a package of sterile gloves.

Now, pin up your hair, if necessary. Then, wash your hands thoroughly.

Note: If you have a beard or very long hair, you'll need to obtain a special sterile disposable cap from the central supply department.

Open the sterile pack along the perforated line and remove the inside package. Place it on a clean, dry surface.

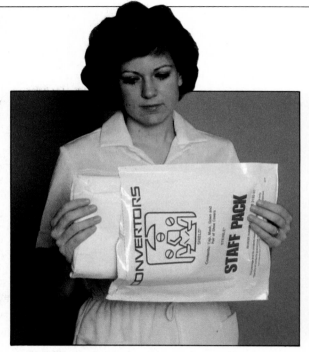

2 To create a sterile field, open the inner package using aseptic technique.

Next, open the package containing the sterile gloves.

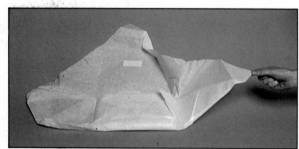

3 Now, with your hands against the insides of the sterile cap, stretch it outward. As you pull the cap downward over your head, gradually remove your hands from inside. Take care not to touch the outside of the cap.

Is all your hair in the cap? If it isn't, carefully tuck your hair inside.

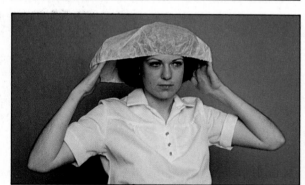

4 Does your hospital require shoe covers? If so, stretch the elasticized shoe cover opening from the inside.

Then, carefully slip the cover over your shoe. Repeat this procedure with the second cover.

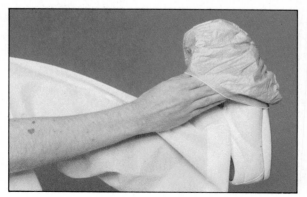

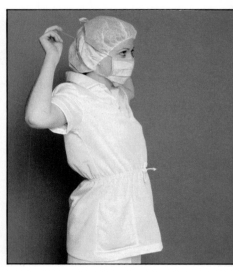

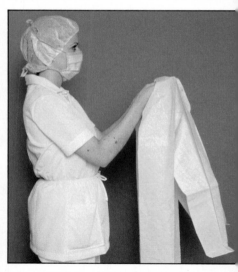

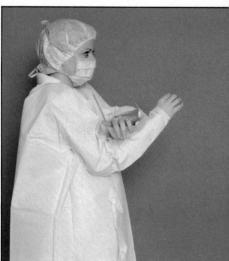

5 Now you're ready to put on your mask. To do this, hold the mask by the top strings and place it over your nose. Tie the strings together, being careful not to contaminate your cap.

Using the bottom strings, pull the mask down. Make sure the mask's bottom edge completely covers your chin. Then, tie the bottom strings.

6 To put on the gown, you'll pick it up from the inside and let it unfold, as the nurse is doing here. Be careful not to let the gown touch anything (including your clothes).

Then, put your hands through the gown's armholes.

7 Hold your arms high and slip both hands into the gown's sleeves, keeping your hands inside the gown. Then, use your left sleeve to pull the right sleeve over your right hand, as shown here. Using the same technique, adjust the left sleeve.

Tie the gown's neck and waist strings. *Note:* The back of the gown's considered contaminated.

Put on your sterile gloves. Then, curve the mask's metal strip over your nose to ensure a proper fit.

How to remove contaminated isolation garb

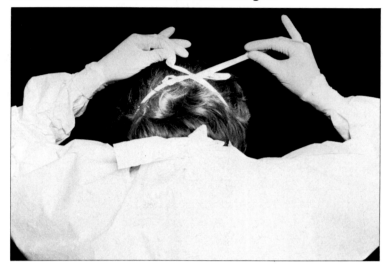

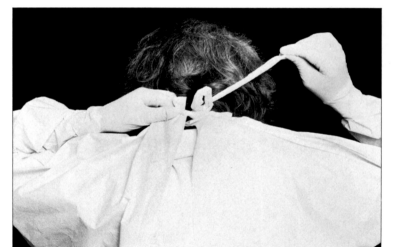

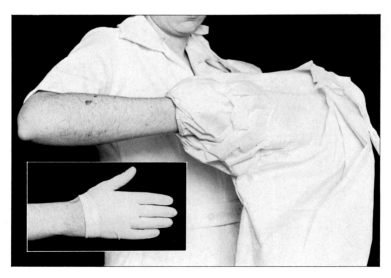

1 *In most cases, you'll remove your isolation garb before leaving a contaminated area. You can prevent cross infection and further contamination by removing your isolation garb properly. Here's how:*

First, untie the mask's bottom strings, then the top strings. Untying the bottom strings first prevents the mask from falling down around your neck. Discard the mask. Then, if you're wearing shoe covers and a cap, remove and discard them.

2 Next, untie the gown's neck strings, as the nurse is doing here. Then, untie the gown's waist strings.

3 Grasp the gown at your left shoulder with your right hand and pull the gown's left side forward and over the glove, as shown here. This will form a cuff on your glove (see inset).

Repeat this procedure with the gown's right side. Be careful not to touch your clothing with the gown or gloves.

Isolation procedures

How to remove contaminated isolation garb continued

4 When you've removed the gown, fold it with the outer contaminated surfaces together, as the nurse is doing here.

Then, roll it into a ball and discard it into your patient's trash receptacle (see inset).

Is the gown nondisposable? If so, place it in the covered linen hamper receptacle.

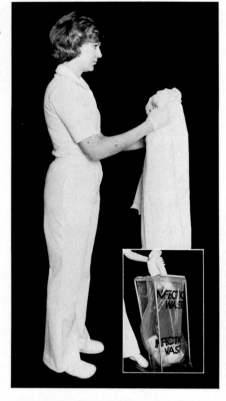

5 Now, place the gloved fingers of your right hand under the cuff of your left glove, as shown here. Inverting the left glove with your right hand, gradually pull off the glove. Discard your left glove in the trash receptacle.

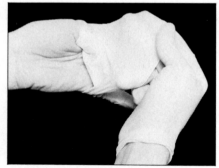

6 Next, use your left hand to grasp the fold of the right glove's cuff. Remove the right glove, as described above, and discard it.

Now, enter the anteroom. Wash your hands with an antiseptic agent and running water.

Suppose your patient's room has no anteroom. Then, clean your hands with the antiseptic agent on the isolation cart. But, don't close the door when leaving the patient's room. Your hands will contaminate the outside door handle. Wash your hands first. Then, close the door.

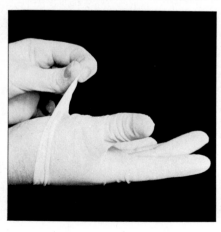

Isolation tips: How to double bag

1 *Imagine you want to remove soiled linens from your patient's isolation room. You'll double bag the linen to help prevent infection from spreading. Here's how:*

Note: You'll adapt this procedure to remove any contaminated article that requires double bagging (such as trash) from any isolation room.

Begin by checking your patient's anteroom (or isolation cart) for the following supplies: clean linen, towel, washcloth, and patient gown; color-coded, moisture-resistant, nylon hamper bag; isolation sticker (if necessary); clean water-soluble bag; and antiseptic cleaning agent.

Then, place a chair near the isolation room door, with the chair's back facing the room. Hang the hamper bag over the back, as shown here.

Put on the necessary isolation garb. Then, take a clean water-soluble bag and the linens into the isolation room.

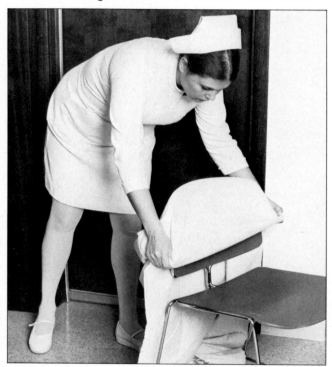

2 Change your patient's bed, putting the soiled linen into the water-soluble bag in the linen covered hamper receptacle.

To prevent any wet towels or washcloths from dissolving the water-soluble bag, wrap dry, soiled linen around the wet pieces.

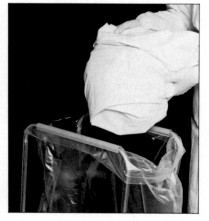

3 When the water-soluble bag's three quarters full, replace it with the clean bag. To do this, remove the filled bag from the linen hamper receptacle, as shown here.

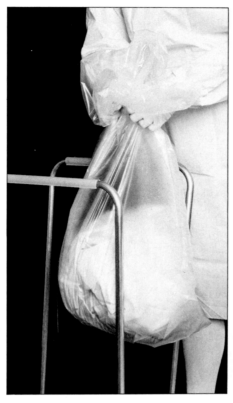

6 Next, place the clean water-soluble bag into the linen hamper. Hang the bag's cuff over the stand's rim.

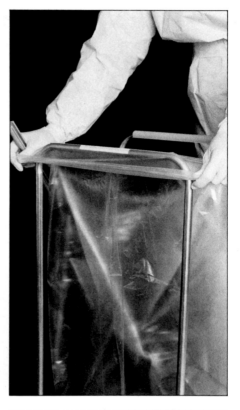

4 Then, pointing the bag's opening away from you, gently push in the sides to expel any air. This prevents the bag from breaking when it's dropped down the laundry chute.

Note: Always replace the water-soluble bag when it's three quarters full or at the end of your shift.

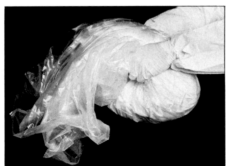

5 Secure the bag's top with the attached plastic tie, as the nurse is doing here.

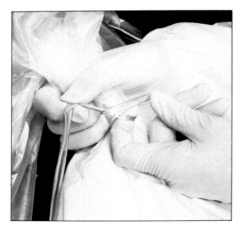

7 As you can see in this photo, you'll put the filled bag upside down into the hamper bag. Then, remove your isolation garb and wash your hands.

To close the hamper bag, pull the tabs under the bag's flap. The flap should invert.

After you complete this part of the procedure, place an isolation identification marker on the bag. Take the bag to the laundry chute. (In some hospitals, housekeeping personnel will pick up the bag after the nurse removes it from the isolation room.)

If a co-worker's available, she can assist you with the double-bagging procedure. However, she'll remain outside the isolation room.

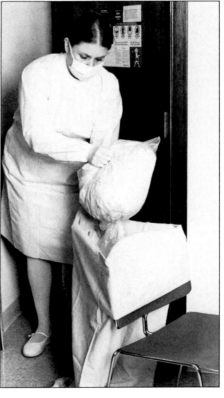

Isolation procedures

How to transport a patient in isolation

1 *Let's assume the doctor orders a lung scan for your patient in isolation. Before bringing her to the X-ray department, you'll need to take certain precautions. Do you know what they are? If you're unsure, this photostory will show you:*

First, notify the X-ray department of your patient's arrival, her state of communicability, and any precautions they need to follow.

Then, bring a clean wheelchair into your patient's anteroom. Holding a clean cotton blanket or sheet diagonally, cover the wheelchair, as shown here.

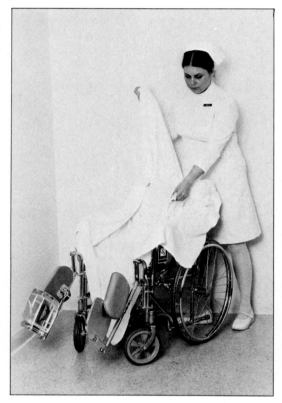
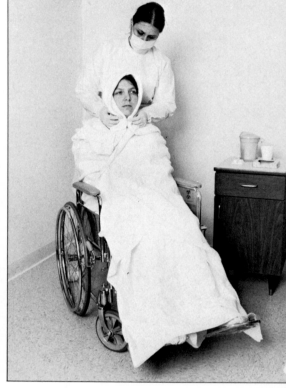

2 Now, put on the necessary isolation garb. Bring the wheelchair into your patient's room, along with an extra set of isolation garb for your patient.

Note: If your patient's in protective isolation, transport her only if absolutely necessary. If she must be transported, you'll need to disinfect the wheelchair before bringing it into the patient's room. Also, bring in sterile isolation garb.

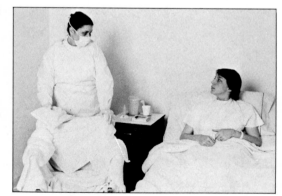

3 Next, explain to your patient what special precautions must be taken before she leaves the room.

Then, put the necessary isolation garb on your patient, using the procedure described on pages 95 and 96.

Remember: If your patient's in respiratory isolation, she'll only need to wear a mask. A patient in wound or skin, or enteric isolation will need to wear a clean isolation gown. Also, place a blanket or incontinent pad on the wheelchair seat and a clean dressing over the infected wound.

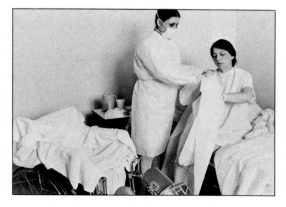
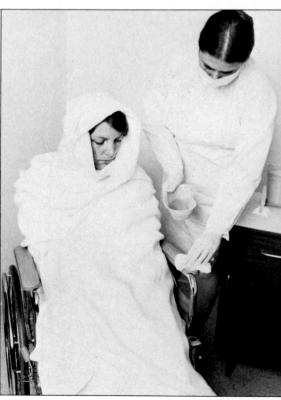

4 Help your patient into the wheelchair. Then, wrap the blanket or sheet around her, as the nurse is doing here. Only your patient's face should be exposed.

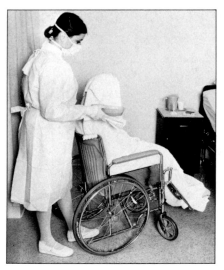

6 When your patient returns from the X-ray department, push the wheelchair just inside the isolation room door.

Then, put on your isolation garb. Pour germicidal solution into an emesis basin. Take the solution and paper towels into the room with you. Push the wheelchair into the isolation room.

7 With your patient still wrapped in the blanket, help her into bed.

Then, remove the blanket and her isolation garb. Discard them into the proper receptacles in the room.

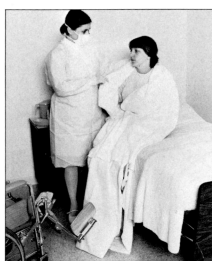

How to terminal clean an isolation room

Whenever a patient in isolation is transferred to another unit or discharged from the hospital, the isolation room and all its contents must be thoroughly cleaned and disinfected. This procedure is known as terminal cleaning. As you know, part of terminal cleaning is a nursing responsibility. You'll need to properly clean, double bag, and remove all supplies from the room before housekeeping completes the terminal cleaning procedure. Although isolation room supplies may vary, here are some guidelines:

• Empty all nondisposable receptacles (such as drainage bottles, urinals and bedpans) into the toilet or sink drain, and wipe them with germicidal solution. If the receptacles are disposable, empty and discard them, according to hospital policy.

• Wipe other patient-care supplies (such as reusable equipment) with a germicidal solution.

• Discard all disposable items into the trash receptacle.

• Strip the bed and place the linen and all other laundry into a water-soluble bag.

• Remove the needle clipper from the needle receptacle and place tape over the receptacle opening.

What about items that can't be double bagged, such as the linen stand or wheelchair? You'll need to wipe them with germicidal solution before removing them from the room. In addition, remember to disinfect equipment that can't be removed from the room; for example, a wall sphygmomanometer holder. But remember, you'll double bag the blood pressure cuff and any respiratory equipment for gas sterilization.

When you've completed your part of terminal cleaning, label all articles CONTAMINATED or ISOLATION. Doing so alerts other hospital employees to follow proper procedures when handling and processing articles, to protect them from contamination. Then, remove the sign from the isolation room door. Finally, send the equipment and supplies to the central supply department, the trash bag to the trash chute room, and the linen bag to the laundry room.

5 Now, before leaving the isolation room, wipe any exposed area on the wheelchair with disinfectant and paper towels.

🖂 *Nursing tip:* Send along an extra set of isolation garb and some impervious bags for use by a staff member in your patient's destination area.

When the person transporting your patient to the X-ray department arrives, push the wheelchair outside the room. Instruct the transporter to tape an isolation card to the wheelchair where it can be seen clearly. If the transporter will have direct contact with your patient, make sure he wears a gown and mask.

Remove your isolation garb and wash your hands.

8 Clean the wheelchair with a paper towel and germicidal solution. Use the paper towel to push the wheelchair into the anteroom.

Finally, remove your isolation garb and wash your hands.

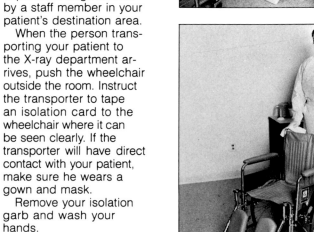

Antibiotic therapy

How much do you know about antibiotic therapy? Suppose you're caring for a patient with a chronic urinary-tract infection caused by gram-negative organisms. If so, he's probably receiving an antibacterial drug that acts directly on the kidneys and bladder.

But what if he isn't responding to this therapy? Do you know what to do next? Read the following pages to learn more about the special nursing implications of antibiotic therapy.

Understanding antibiotics

Before we discuss antibiotic therapy, we have to consider antibiotics. What exactly is an antibiotic? It's a chemical substance—produced by microorganisms—that inhibits or destroys the growth of other microorganisms. An antibiotic that inhibits microorganism growth is called *bacteriostatic*. An antibiotic that destroys microorganism growth is called *bactericidal*.

Antibiotics can be classified in several ways. But, as a nurse, you're probably most familiar with classification by antimicrobial activity. Using this classification system, three main types of antibiotics exist:
• narrow spectrum: a drug effective against gram-positive cocci and bacteria; for example, penicillin G
• broad spectrum: a drug effective against gram-positive cocci and gram-negative bacilli; for example, cephalosporin
• drugs effective against aerobic gram-negative bacilli; for example, aminoglycosides.

To ensure maximum antibiotic effectiveness against a specific organism, you'll also need to know:
• location of infection
• correct administration route for drug
• drug's effectiveness against foreign matter, such as pus or calculi
• route by which drug is excreted.

The doctor may order two or more antibiotics administered simultaneously. This antibiotic therapy is usually used when the patient has a mixed bacterial infection caused by two or more microorganisms, or a life-threatening infection caused by an unidentified microorganism. He may also order antibiotics administered simultaneously when he wants to enhance the antibacterial activity of one or both antibiotics, or to prevent the emergence of resistant microorganisms.

Nurses' guide to common antibiotics

The best way to avoid antibiotic complications is to learn about the drugs *before* starting therapy. Learn how they work and why certain ones are chosen. Otherwise, you may face a variety of unexpected problems. For your reference, here's a list of commonly administered antibiotics. For more information on these and other antibiotics, refer to the NURSE'S GUIDE TO DRUGS™, or the NURSE'S DRUG HANDBOOK™, by Intermed Communications, Inc.

Penicillin G potassium
Novopen-G*

Classification
Penicillin that is bactericidal for many gram-positive and gram-negative microorganisms

Indications
Moderate to severe systemic infections

Precautions
Use cautiously in patients with other drug allergies, especially to cephalosporins (possible cross-allergenicity).

Side effects
Hemolytic anemia, leukopenia, thrombocytopenia, neuropathy, arthralgia, prostration, possible severe to fatal potassium poisoning with high doses (hyperreflexia, convulsions, coma), hypersensitivity (rash, urticaria, maculo-papular eruptions, exfoliative dermatitis, chills, fever, edema, anaphylaxis), overgrowth of nonsusceptible organisms

Dose
Adults:
1.6 to 3.2 million units P.O. daily, divided into doses given every 6 hours (1 mg = 1,600 units); 1.2 to 24 million units I.M. or I.V. daily, in equal doses given every 4 hours
Children under age 12:
25,000 to 100,000 units/kg P.O. daily divided into doses given every 6 hours; or 25,000 to 300,000 units/kg I.M. or I.V. daily, divided into doses given every 4 hours

Interactions
Chloramphenicol, erythromycin, tetracycline:
Antibiotic antagonism. Give penicillin at least 1 hour before bacteriostatic antibiotics.
Probenecid:
Increased blood levels of penicillin. Probenecid is often used for this purpose.

Nursing considerations
• If possible, obtain cultures for sensitivity tests before starting therapy. Not necessary to wait for culture and sensitivity results before beginning therapy.
• Before giving penicillin, ask patient if he's had any previous allergic reactions to this drug. However, a negative history of penicillin allergy is no guarantee against a future allergic reaction.
• Tell patient to call the doctor if he develops rash, fever, or chills. A rash is the most common allergic reaction.
• Be prepared for possible allergic reaction to this drug. Have available emergency equipment and medications needed for resuscitation.
• Instruct patient to take medication exactly as prescribed, even if he feels better. Schedule dosages evenly throughout each 24-hour period.
• When given orally, drug may cause GI disturbances. Food may interfere with drug absorption, so give 1 to 2 hours before meals or 2 to 3 hours after.
• Don't give I.M. or I.V. unless infection is severe or patient can't take oral dose. Extremely painful when given I.M.
• Check complete blood cell (CBC) count and transaminase levels frequently. Drug may cause leukopenia, thrombocytopenia, and elevated serum glutamic-oxaloacetic transaminase (SGOT) and serum glutamic-pyruvic transaminase (SGPT) levels.
• If patient has high serum level of this drug, he may have convulsions. Be prepared by keeping side rails up on bed and padded tongue blade handy.
• When giving I.V., mix drug with 5% dextrose in water or normal saline solution. Don't mix with other solutions; they may prove incompatible.
• Give drug I.V. intermittently to prevent vein irritation. Change site every 24 to 48 hours.
• Large doses may cause increased yeast growths. Urge patient to report signs and symptoms to you or his doctor, especially *Candida* vaginal infections in females.
• Observe patient closely with prolonged therapy; other superinfections may occur, especially in patients who are elderly, debilitated, or have low resistance to infection from immunosuppressive drug therapy or radiation.
• Monitor serum potassium levels.
• Check drug's expiration date. Warn patient never to use leftover penicillin tablets for a new illness or to share penicillin with family and friends.

*Available in both the United States and in Canada

Sulfisoxazole
Gantrisin*

Classification
Sulfonamide effectively treats susceptible gram-positive and gram-negative bacteria.

Indications
Urinary tract and systemic infections

Precautions
Contraindicated in porphyria and in infants less than 2 months old (except in congenital toxoplasmosis). Use cautiously in patients with impaired hepatic or renal function, severe allergy, or bronchial asthma, and glucose-6-Phosphate Dehydrogenase (G-6 PD) deficiency.

Side effects
Agranulocytosis, aplastic anemia, thrombocytopenia, leukopenia, megaloblastic anemia, hemolytic anemia, purpura, headache, mental depression, convulsions, hallucinations, nausea, vomiting, diarrhea, abdominal pain, anorexia, stomatitis, toxic nephrosis with oliguria and anuria, crystalluria, hematuria, erythema multiforme (Stevens-Johnson syndrome), generalized skin eruption, epidermal necrolysis, urticaria, pruritus, exfoliative dermatitis, photosensitization, serum sickness, drug fever, chills

Dose
Adults:
Initially, 2 to 4 grams P.O., then 1 to 2 grams P.O. four times a day; extended-release suspension 4 to 5 grams P.O. every 12 hours
Children over 2 months:
Initially, 75 mg/kg P.O. daily or 2 gm/m² P.O. daily in equal doses every 6 hours; then 150 mg/kg or 4 gm/m² P.O. daily in equal doses every 6 hours; extended-release suspension 60 to 70 mg/kg P.O. every 12 hours
Adults and children over 2 months:
Parenteral dosages (sulfisoxazole diolamine) initially, 50 mg/kg or 1 .125 gm/m² by slow I.V. injection, then 100 mg/kg daily or 2.25 gm/m² daily in equal doses every 6 hours by slow I.V. injection

Interactions
PABA-containing local anesthetics and other PABA drugs: Inhibited antibacterial action. Don't use together.
Ammonium chloride, ascorbic acid, paraldehyde: Doses sufficient to acidify urine may cause crystalluria and precipitation of sulfonamide. Don't use together.

Nursing considerations
• Tell patient to drink 8 oz. water with each dose and to drink plenty of water throughout the day to prevent crystalluria. Monitor fluid intake and urinary output. Intake should be sufficient to produce output of 1,500 ml daily. To help prevent crystalluria, doctor may order sodium bicarbonate to alkalinize urine.
• Tell patient to take medication for as long as prescribed, even if he feels better. Warn patient to avoid direct sunlight and ultraviolet light to prevent photosensitivity reaction.
• Monitor urinary cultures and sensitivities, CBC, and urinalysis before and during therapy.
• Parenteral form of drug (sulfisoxale diolamine) can be given I.M. or subcutaneously, but these routes are discouraged. Intravenous administration not recommended.
• Diluents other than sterile distilled water may cause precipitation.
• Tell patient to report early signs of blood dyscrasias immediately, and discontinue drug.
• During long-term therapy, watch for signs of GI superinfection.
• When given preoperatively, the patient should receive a low-residue diet and as few enemas and cathartics as possible.
• Vitamin K₁ may reverse sulfonamide-induced hypoprothrombinemia.

Cephalothin sodium
(Keflin Neutral*)

Classification
Cephalosporin (semisynthetic) that is effective against most gram-positive and some gram-negative organisms

Indications
Treatment of serious infections of respiratory, genitourinary, or gastrointestinal tract; skin and soft tissue infections (including peritonitis); bone and joint infections; septicemia; endocarditis; and meningitis from *E. coli* and other coliform bacteria, Enterobacteriaceae, enterococci, gonococci, *H. influenzae, Klebsiella, P. mirabilis, Salmonella, S. aureus, Shigella, S. pneumoniae, Staphylococci,* and *S. viridens*

Precautions
Use cautiously in patients with impaired renal function and in those with history of sensitivity to penicillin. Before administering first dose, ask patient if he's had any reaction to previous cephalosporin or penicillin therapy.

Side effects
Hemolytic anemia, headache, malaise, paresthesias, dizziness, nausea, anorexia, vomiting, diarrhea, glossitis, dyspepsia, abdominal cramps, tenesmus, anal pruritus, oral candidiasis (thrush), genital pruritus and moniliasis, maculopapular and erythematous rashes, urticaria, hypersensitivity, dyspnea

Dose
Adults
500 mg to 1 gram I.M. or I.V. (or intraperitoneally) every 4 to 6 hours; in life-threatening infections, up to 2 grams every 4 hours
Children under 12 years:
14 to 27 mg/kg I.V. every 4 hours, or 20 to 40 mg/kg every 6 hours; dose should be proportionately less in accordance with age, weight, and severity of infection.

Interactions
Probenecid:
Use cautiously; increases blood levels of cephalosporins.

Nursing considerations
• Obtain cultures for sensitivity tests before beginning therapy, but therapy may begin pending results of cultures and sensitivity tests.
• Watch for superinfection. Prolonged use may result in overgrowth of nonsusceptible organisms.
• To prevent undue pain, avoid administering I.M., if possible.
• When giving I.V., check frequently for vein irritation and phlebitis. Alternate injection sites if I.V. therapy lasts longer than 3 days.
• Administer urine glucose tests with Benedict's Qualitative Reagent, Clinitest, or Fehling's solution. These may give false positive solution during cephalosporin therapy. Clinistix, Diastix, and Tes-Tape are not affected.

Tetracycline hydrochloride
(Achromycin*)

Classification
Tetracycline that is effective against gram-positive and gram-negative bacteria

Indications
Rickettsia diseases and infections caused by sensitive gram-negative and gram-positive organisms, trachoma, amebiasis (with amebicide)

Precautions
Use with extreme caution in patients with impaired renal or hepatic function. Use during last half of pregnancy and in children younger than age 8 may cause permanent discoloration of teeth, enamel defects, and retardation of bone growth.

Side effects
Neutropenia, eosinophilia, pericarditis, sore throat, glossitis, dysphagia, anorexia, nausea, vomiting, diarrhea, enterocolitis, anogenital inflammatory irritation after I.M. injection, increased BUN, diabetes insipidus syndrome, maculopapular and erythematous rashes, urticaria, photosensitivity, increased pigmentation, hypersensitivity

Dose
Adults:
250 to 500 mg P.O. every 6 hours; 250 mg I.M. daily or 150 mg I.M. every 12 hours; or 250 to 500 mg I.V. every 8 to 12 hours (I.M. and I.V. hydrochloride salt only)
Children over age 8:
25 to 50 mg/kg P.O. daily in equal doses every 6 hours; 15 to 25 mg/kg/day (maximum 250 mg) I.M. single dose or in equal doses every 8 to 12 hours; or 10 to 20 mg/kg I.V. daily, in equal doses every 12 hours

Interactions
Antacids (including NaHCO₃) and laxatives containing aluminum, magnesium, or calcium; food, and dairy products: decreased antibiotic absorption. Give antibiotic 1 hour before or 2 hours after any of the above.
Ferrous sulfate and other iron products; zinc: decreased antibiotic absorption. Give tetracyclines 3 hours after or 2 hours before iron administration.
Methoxyflurane:
May cause severe nephrotoxicity with tetracyclines. Monitor carefully.

Nursing considerations
• Obtain cultures for sensitivity tests before starting therapy, if possible.
• Tell patient that drug effectiveness is reduced when taken with dairy products, food, antacids, or iron products.
• Instruct patient to take each dose with 8 oz. of water on an empty stomach, at least 1 hour before meals or 2 hours afterward. Give at least 1 hour before bedtime to prevent esophagitis.
• Avoid extravasation. Patient may develop thrombophlebitis with I.V. administration.
• Check drug's expiration date. Outdated or deteriorated tetracycline may cause nephrotoxicity.
• Discard I.M. solutions after 24 hours because they deteriorate. However, discard Achromycin solution in 12 hours.
• Do not expose drugs to light or heat.
• Inject I.M. dosage deeply. Warn patient that it may be painful. Rotate sites. I.M. preparations often contain a local anesthetic; ask patient about hypersensitivity to local anesthetics.
• Watch for overgrowth of nonsensitive organisms. Check patient's tongue for infection. Stress good oral hygiene. If superinfection occurs, drug should be discontinued.
• Tell patient to take medication exactly as prescribed, even if he feels better. Streptococcal infections must be treated for at least 10 days.

Antibiotic therapy

Nurses' guide to common antibiotics continued

Vancomycin hydrochloride
(Vancocin*)

Classification
Effective against gram-positive bacteria

Indications
Severe staphylococcal infections when other antibiotics are ineffective or contraindicated

Precautions
Contraindicated in patients receiving other neurotoxic, nephrotoxic, or ototoxic drugs. Use cautiously in patients with impaired hepatic and renal function; also with preexisting hearing loss; in patients over age 60; and in patients with allergies to other antibiotics.

Side effects
Transient eosinophilia, tinnitus, ototoxicity, nausea, nephrotoxicity, pain or thrombophlebitis with I.V. administration, chills, fever, anaphylaxis, overgrowth of nonsusceptible organisms

Dose
Adults:
500 mg I.V. every 6 hours or 1 gram every 12 hours
Children under age 12:
44 mg/kg I.V. daily, in equal doses every 6 hours
Neonates:
10 mg/kg I.V. daily, in equal doses every 6 to 12 hours
Staphylococcal enterocolitis
Adults:
500 mg P.O. in 30 ml water every 6 hours
Children under age 12:
44 mg/kg P.O. daily, divided every 6 hours in 30 ml water

Interactions
None significant

Nursing considerations
• Tell patient to take medication exactly as directed, even if he feels better. Patient with staphylococcal endocarditis must take drug at least 3 weeks.
• Patients should receive auditory function tests before and during therapy. If ringing in ears occurs, stop drug immediately.
• Do not give drug I.M.
• For I.V. infusion, dilute drug in 200 ml solution and infuse over 20 to 30 minutes. Check site daily for phlebitis and irritation. Report pain at infusion site. Avoid extravasation to prevent tissue irritation and necrosis.
• Monitor renal function (BUN, serum creatinine, urinalysis, creatinine clearance, urinary output) before and during therapy. Watch for signs of superinfection.
• Refrigerate I.V. solution after reconstitution and use within 96 hours.
• Oral preparation remains stable for 2 weeks, if refrigerated.
• Drug has been used recently to treat pseudomembranous colitis caused by clindamycin.
• Culture and sensitivity tests should be performed before first dose, if possible.
• During therapy, check that patient has routine hematologic studies, urinalysis, and liver and renal function studies.
• Instruct patient to report any side effects.

Gentamicin sulfate
(Garamycin*)

Classification:
Aminoglycosides affect the properties for many serious gram-negative bacillary infections.

Indications
Serious infections caused by sensitive *Pseudomonas aeruginosa, Escherichia coli, Proteus, Klebsiella, Serratia, Enterobacter, Citrobacter, Staphylococcus* species

Precautions
Use cautiously in patients with impaired renal function; in neonates, infants, and elderly patients.

Side effects
Headache, lethargy, organic brain syndrome, ototoxicity (tinnitus, vertigo, roaring in the ears, hearing loss), nausea, vomiting, nephrotoxicity, rash, urticaria

Dose
Adults with normal renal function:
3 mg/kg/day in equal doses every 8 hours I.M. or I.V. infusion (in 50 to 200 ml of normal saline solution or 5% dextrose in water infused over 30 minutes to 2 hours); for life-threatening infections, patient may receive up to 5 mg/kg/day in 3 to 4 equal dosages.
Children under 12 years with normal renal function:
2 to 2.5 mg/kg I.M. or I.V. infusion every 8 hours
Infants and neonates over 1 week with normal renal function:
2.5 mg/kg every 8 hours I.M. or I.V. infusion
Neonates under 1 week:
2.5 mg/kg I.V. every 12 hours. For I.V. infusion, dilute in normal saline solution or 5% dextrose in water and infuse over ½ to 2 hours.

Interactions
Ethacrynic acid, furosemide:
Increased ototoxicity. Use cautiously.
Dimenhydrinate:
Use cautiously, may mask ototoxicity symptoms.
Carbenicillin:
Schedule doses 1 hour apart from gentamicin sulfate. Don't mix together in I.V.
Cephalosporins:
Use cautiously; increases nephrotoxicity.
Other aminoglycosides, methoxyflurane:
Use cautiously; increases ototoxicity and nephrotoxcity.

Nursing considerations
• Obtain specimen for culture and sensitivity before first dose, if possible. Therapy may begin pending test results.
• Weigh patient and obtain baseline renal function studies before therapy begins.
• Monitor renal function (output, specific gravity, urinalysis, blood urea nitrogen, creatine). Notify doctor of decreasing renal function.
• Keep patient well hydrated while taking this drug.
• Evaluate patient's hearing before and during therapy. Notify doctor if patient complains of tinnitus, vertigo, hearing loss.
• Watch for superinfection (continued fever and other signs of new infections, especially of upper respiratory tract).
• Obtain specimen for gentamicin blood levels ½ hour before and 1 hour after dose. Tell lab if patient is also taking carbenicillin or other antibiotic.
• Usual duration of therapy is 7 to 10 days. If no response in 3 to 5 days, therapy should be stopped and new specimens obtained for culture and sensitivity.
• After completing I.V. infusion, flush line with normal saline solution to remove any remaining drug.
• In case of overdose or toxic reaction, hemodialysis aids in drug removal.

Chloramphenicol
Chloramphenicol palmitate, chloramphenicol sodium succinate
(Chloromycetin*)

Classification
Miscellaneous. (Drug has bacteriostatic or bactericidal effect on a variety of infective agents, primarily bacterial and viral.)

Indications
Hemophilus influenzae meningitis, severe infections caused by sensitive *Salmonella* species including *S. typhi* infection, *Rickettsia*, lymphogranuloma, psittacosis, various sensitive gram-negative organisms causing meningitis, bacteremia, or other serious infections

Precautions
Use cautiously in patients with impaired hepatic or renal function, or with other drugs causing bone marrow disease or blood disorders. Don't use for infections susceptible to other agents or for trivial infections, such as colds.

Side effects
Aplastic anemia, hypoplastic anemia, granulocytopenia, thrombocytopenia, headache, mild depression, confusion, delirium, peripheral neuropathy with prolonged therapy, optic neuritis (in cystic fibrosis patients), glossitis, decreased visual acuity, nausea, vomiting, stomatitis, diarrhea, enterocolitis, infections by nonsusceptible organisms, hypersensitivity reaction (fever, rash, urticaria, anaphylaxis), gray baby syndrome (abdominal distension, cyanosis, vasomotor collapse, death within a few hours of onset of symptoms)

Dose
Adults and children under age 12:
50 to 100 mg/kg P.O. or I.V. daily, in equal doses every 6 hours. Maximum dose is 100 mg/kg daily.
Premature infants and neonates (2 weeks or younger):
25 mg/kg P.O. or I.V. daily, in equal doses every 6 hours. I.V. route must be used to treat meningitis.

Interactions
Penicillins:
Antagonized antibacterial effect. Give penicillin at least 1 hour before or after drug administration.
Acetaminophen:
Elevated chloramphenicol levels. Monitor for toxicity.
Anticoagulants and Phenytoin sodium (Dilantin):*
Use cautiously.

Nursing considerations
• Culture and sensitivity tests should be done initially, and as needed. Therapy may begin pending test results.
• Monitor CBC count, platelets, serum iron levels, and reticulocytes before and every 2 days during therapy. Stop drug immediately if anemia, reticulocytopenia, leukopenia, or thrombocytopenia develops.
• Give I.V. slowly over 1 minute. Check injection site daily for phlebitis and irritation.
• Instruct patient to report side effects, especially nausea, vomiting, diarrhea, fever, confusion, sore throat, or mouth sores.
• Reconstitute one gram vial of powder with 10 ml sterile water for injection. Concentration will be 100 mg/ml.
• Tell patient to take medication for as long as prescribed, exactly as directed, even if he feels better.
• When reconstituted, solution remains stable at room temperature for 30 days. Refrigeration is recommended, however. Discard solution if cloudy.

*Available in both the United States and in Canada

Erythromycin

Erythromycin base
(E-Mycin*)
Erythromycin estolate
(Ilosone*)
Erythromycin ethylsuccinate
(E.E.S.)

Erythromycin gluceptate
(Ilotycin*)
Erythromycin lactobionate
(Erythrocin*)
Erythromycin stearate
(Bristamycin)

Classification
Miscellaneous. (Drug has a bacteriostatic or bactericidal effect on a variety of infective agents, primarily bacterial and viral.)

Indications
Acute pelvic inflammatory disease caused by *Neisseria gonorrhoeae* and Legionnaire's disease

Precautions
Use cautiously in impaired hepatic function.

Side effects
Abdominal pain and cramping, nausea, vomiting, diarrhea, venous irritation, thrombophlebitis following I.V. injection, urticaria, rashes, overgrowth of nonsusceptible bacteria or fungi, anaphylaxis, fever, cholestatic hepatitis (with erthromycin estolate)

Dose
Women:
Initially, 500 mg I.V. (erythromycin gluceptate, lactobionate) every 6 hours for 3 days, then 250 mg (erythromycin base, estolate, stearate) or 400 mg (erythromycin ethylsuccinate) P.O. every 6 hours for 7 days
Endocarditis prophylaxis, for dental procedures:
Adults:
500 mg (erythromycin base, estolate, stearate) P.O. before procedure, followed by 250 mg P.O. every 6 hours for 4 doses afterward; or 1,200 mg (erythromycin ethylsuccinate) P.O. before procedure, followed by 400 mg P.O. every 6 hours for 4 doses afterward
Children:
30 to 50 mg/kg (oral erythromycin salts) P.O. daily in equal doses every 6 hours. Give 1 dose before procedure and 4 doses afterward.
Mild to moderately severe respiratory tract, skin and soft-tissue infections caused by sensitive group A beta-hemolytic streptococci, Diplococci pneumoniae, Mycoplasma pneumoniae, Corynebacterium diphtheriae, Bordetella pertussis, Listeria monocytogenes
Adults:
250 mg to 500 mg (erythromycin base, estolate, stearate) P.O. every 6 hours; or 400 to 800 mg (erythromycin ethylsuccinate) P.O. every 6 hours; or 15 to 20 mg/kg I.V. daily, as continuous infusion or divided every 6 hours
Children:
30 to 50 mg/kg (oral erythromycin salts) P.O. daily, divided every 6 hours; or 15 to 20 mg/kg I.V. daily, divided every 4 to 6 hours
Syphilis
Adults:
500 mg (erythromycin base, estolate, stearate) P.O. four times daily for 15 days

Interactions
Clindamycin, lincomycin:
May be antagonistic. Don't use together.
Penicillins:
Antagonized antibacterial effect. Give penicillin at least 1 hour before.

Nursing considerations
• Culture and sensitivity tests should be performed initially, and as ordered.
• For best absorption, instruct patient to take oral form of drug with 8 oz. of water 1 hour before or 2 hours after meals. Patient may take coated tablets with meals. Warn patient not to drink fruit juice with medication. Chewable erythromycin tablets should not be swallowed whole.
• Drug may cause an overgrowth of nonsusceptible bacteria or fungi. Watch for signs and symptoms of superinfections.
• Tell patient to take medication for as long as prescribed, exactly as directed, even if he feels better. Streptococcal infections should be treated for 10 days.
• Instruct patient to report any side effects, especially nausea, abdominal pain, or fever.
• Administer I.V. dose over 20 to 60 minutes. Dilute each 250 mg in at least 100 ml 5% dextrose in water or normal saline solution.

Administering antibiotics: Some guidelines

The doctor will choose antibiotic therapy for your patient based on the patient's history, condition, clinical situation, and available microbiologic information.

However, the key to the effectiveness of antibiotic therapy is you. You must obtain a quality specimen for culture, administer the proper amount of prescribed antibiotic at the right time, and closely monitor your patient for signs of improvement.

So whenever antibiotic therapy is ordered, follow these guidelines:
• Obtain an accurate patient history, including his age, weight, height, allergies, past reactions to drugs, and current lab findings—especially hepatic and renal function.
• Time drug administration carefully. In some cases, giving an oral drug during or shortly after mealtime may decrease drug absorption. Also, oral penicillin and tetracyclines should not be given at mealtime, because certain foods inactivate them. If you want to know more about the effect of food on specific antibiotics, check with your hospital's pharmacy or refer to the NURSE'S DRUG HANDBOOK™, *Intermed Communications, Inc.*
• Monitor your patient for side effects, especially signs of an allergic reaction, such as fever, rash, and dyspnea. If present, notify the doctor. Also watch for signs and symptoms of anaphylactic shock. Be prepared to administer epinephrine hydrochloride (Sus-Phrine*), as ordered.
• Support the patient's own defense mechanisms by promoting proper rest, nutrition, fluid intake, and ensure good hygiene.
• Check for signs of superinfection, especially in the patient's mouth, pharynx, lungs, and vagina. Localized signs and symptoms include redness, itching, and swelling. Systemic signs of superinfection include fever. If you observe any of these, notify the doctor promptly.
• Tell your patient to take prescribed medication as directed, even if he feels better.

Learning about resistant microorganisms

Antibiotic drugs are rapidly becoming the most commonly prescribed medications in health care. And, because of their frequent use, misuse, and overuse, microorganisms resistant to antibiotics are becoming increasingly common. As you probably know, resistant microorganisms may cause nosocomial infections.

No wonder, then, that administering antibiotics imposes a big responsibility on you. But, you're already aware of that because of the special antibiotic precautions hospitals take. Several hospitals, for example, have committees to monitor antibiotic use, including limiting the time periods antibiotic orders are valid. Other hospitals maintain a reserve of certain antibiotics to prescribe for those emergencies in which a causative microorganism is antibiotic resistant.

Follow these guidelines to prevent resistant microorganisms:
• Maintain strict aseptic technique when administering antibiotics.
• Closely monitor your patient's culture and sensitivity test results. Notify the doctor if the test results don't support the use of the prescribed antibiotics.
• Carefully assess your patient's condition daily.
• Accurately document all antibiotic therapy.

How many antibiotic misuses can you name? Some common ones are:
• prescribing antibiotics to treat infections and fevers before determining causative microorganism
• prescribing ineffective antibiotic dosage.
• relying on antibiotics alone when surgical drainage is indicated
• keeping patient on antibiotic therapy when the microorganisms are known to be resistant to the drugs.
• failing to adequately remove spilled antibiotics, or inadvertently squirting parenteral antibiotics into the air, causing airborne microorganisms to become drug resistant.

If you see any of these antibiotic misuses or overuses, document the incident and contact your hospital's infection-control practitioner for further action.

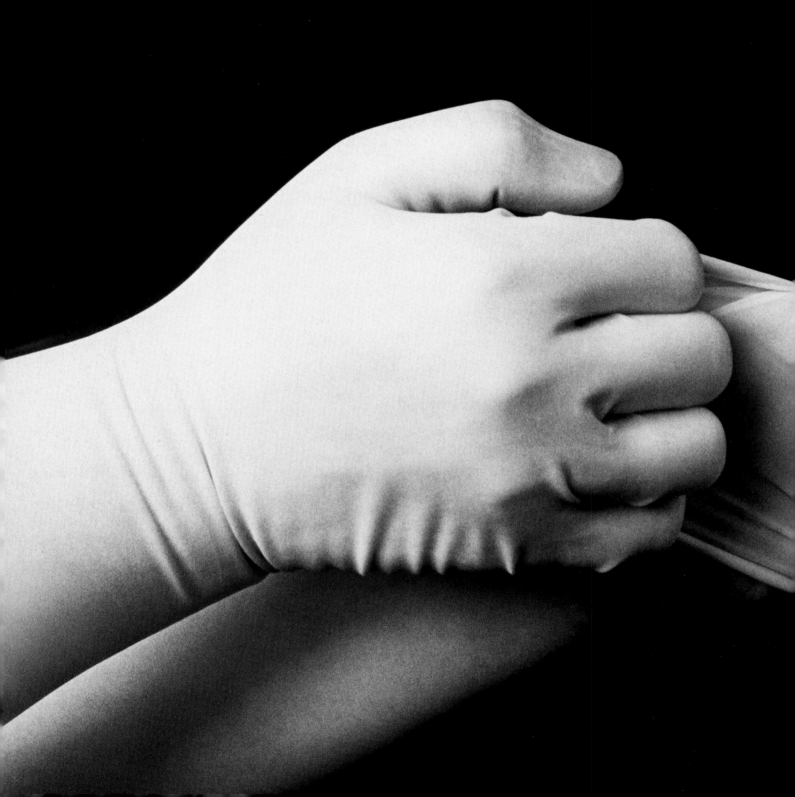

Coping with Invasive Therapy

Percutaneous pathways

Surgical wounds

External body openings

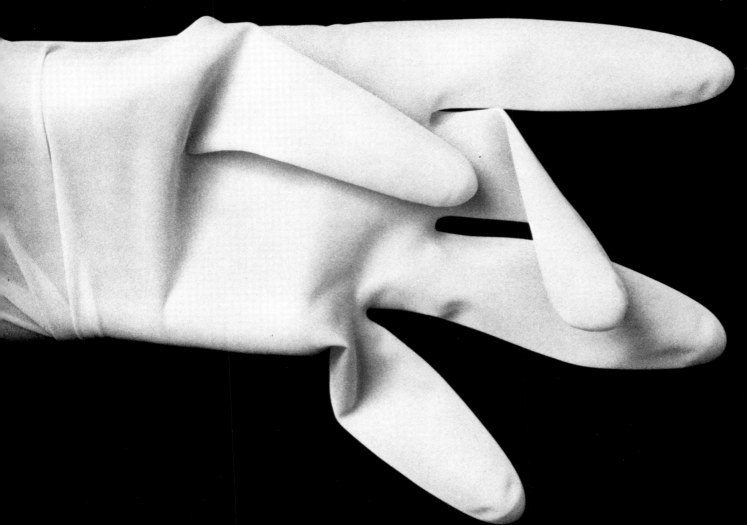

Percutaneous pathways

Controlling infection while caring for a patient with an I.V. line in place plays a major role in your nursing responsibilities. Over the next few pages, we'll show you how to maintain proper aseptic technique while:
• preparing your patient's skin for needle or catheter insertion
• performing venipuncture
• adding a medication to an I.V. solution
• changing the dressing on a central venous pressure (CVP) line.

In addition, we'll explain how using an I.V. filter minimizes the risk of infection, and why some I.V. procedures carry more risks than others.

Read over these pages carefully.

Preventing I.V.-associated infections: Some guidelines

Intravenous therapy poses a potential infection risk to a patient. But, by taking special precautions, you can help reduce this risk.

Preventing development of an infection is always easier than curing an existing one.

When caring for any patient on I.V. therapy, follow these guidelines:
• Always use strict aseptic technique during an I.V. insertion, when adding medications, and when changing I.V. tubing or dressings. If a needle or catheter is inserted during an emergency, without proper aseptic technique, remove and restart the I.V. as soon as the patient's condition stabilizes.
• Before administering any I.V. solution, check the solution for turbidity or precipitate. Examine the bottle or bag for cracks, leaks, or punctures. If you see any of the above, discard the I.V. solution and container. Also, discard any I.V. container with a broken seal, or return it to the hospital pharmacy.
• Examine the needle or catheter for barbs or roughness on the bevel, or errors in labeling or packaging. If you're using a catheter, check the tip for frayed edges.
• Next, clean the site you've chosen for insertion with iodophor solution, unless your patient's allergic to iodine. In this case, use alcohol.
• After you've performed venipuncture, make sure the needle and catheter are secured to your patient's skin, to prevent microorganisms from entering the insertion site.
• Administer all I.V. solutions immediately after opening or within 24 hours. Label the bottle with your patient's name, any added medications, and time of mixing and hanging. Discard an I.V. solution with added medications after 24 hours.
• Examine the I.V. insertion site daily for signs of infection or infiltration; for example, edema, redness, warmth, tenderness, or discharge. Change the needle or catheter every 48 to 72 hours, using a different vein. If you see signs of subcutaneous infiltration, change the needle and catheter immediately.
• Change the I.V. tubing and dressing every 24 to 48 hours, following your hospital's policy. During the dressing change, clean the insertion area with an iodophor solution, unless your patient's allergic to iodine. Apply an antimicrobial ointment at the insertion site.

Using aseptic technique

Although the infection risks of I.V. therapy may be difficult to eliminate, you can help minimize them by maintaining aseptic technique during all I.V. procedures. To begin, always wash your hands thoroughly. Avoid wearing nail polish; even the smallest cracks in polish may carry microorganisms. Also, nail polish may flake off your nails and contaminate I.V. equipment.

When necessary (or according to your hospital's policy), wear a mask and sterile gloves. Make sure you put them on correctly without contaminating the outside surfaces. If you must lower the mask around your neck during the procedure, discard and replace it.

Use only sterile equipment. Before opening equipment packages, check for holes, tears, or punctures. Also, check expiration dates. If you'll be wearing sterile gloves during the procedure, remember to open and prepare all your supplies before putting them on. Be very careful not to contaminate your equipment at any time before or during the procedure.

Understanding percutaneous procedures

Whenever you insert a needle, catheter, or wire into your patient's skin, you're performing a percutaneous procedure. And any percutaneous procedure may increase your patient's potential for infection. Why? Because the puncture caused by the needle, catheter, or wire allows microorganisms on the insertion device or his skin to enter his body.

Of course, the longer the device remains in place, the greater the risk of infection. So, when the insertion device is removed immediately after the procedure, the infection risk is *short-term*. (Thoracentesis and a subcutaneous injection are both short-term percutaneous procedures.)

But, when the insertion device remains in the skin for some time after the procedure, the infection risk is *long-term*. (Central I.V. lines and external cardiac pacemakers are examples of long-term percutaneous procedures.)

In many cases, long-term procedures also involve I.V. tubing, solution, additives, and bottles, which provide additional contamination sources not found in short-term procedures.

How to prep your patient's skin

1 *Preparing your patient's skin, usually called prepping, is essential to reduce the infection risk of I.V. therapy. Why? Because prepping destroys microorganisms on the skin's surface that may otherwise enter through the insertion site. Follow these steps to properly prep your patient's skin:*

First, make sure you have the necessary equipment: an antiseptic agent, such as an iodine preparation or iodophor solution; alcohol wipes; and 4"x4" sterile gauze pads (if needed).

Important: If your patient's allergic to iodine, use 70% alcohol.

Does the doctor want the area cleaned before applying the antiseptic? If so, use a cleaning agent, such as pHisoHex.

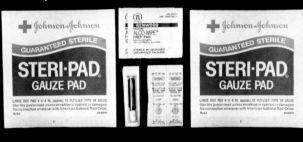

3 Now, clean the insertion area with antiseptic agent. To do this, begin at the intended insertion site and work outward in an area about 2" (5.1 cm) in diameter. Repeat this procedure three times, using a clean antiseptic swab each time.

Allow the antiseptic to dry for at least 30 seconds before proceeding with the insertion. Never wave your hands over the skin to dry it. Doing so may contaminate the area.

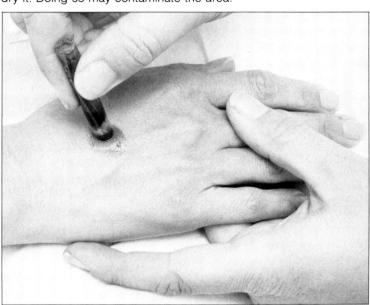

2 Now, wash your hands thoroughly. Explain the procedure to your patient and expose the insertion area.

If your patient has a lot of hair on the site you've selected for insertion, shave the area *around* it. *Never* shave directly over the insertion site.

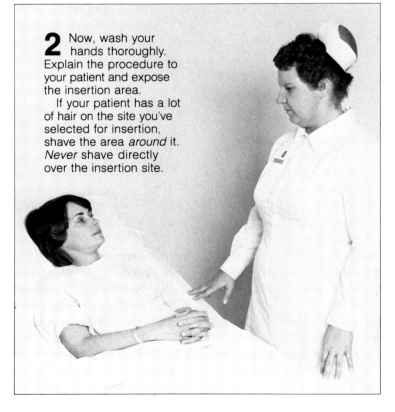

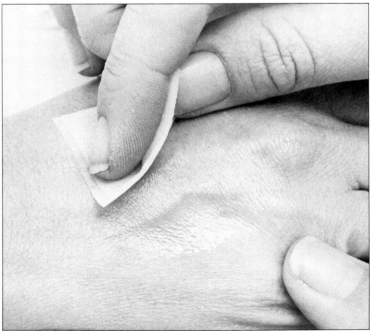

4 Are you using an iodine preparation? In this case, you may need to wipe off the antiseptic with alcohol to better visualize your patient's vein.

If you must palpate your patient's vein again, be sure to put on sterile gloves.

Percutaneous pathways

Inserting a peripheral line using a winged-tip needle

1 *Let's say 30-year-old Andrea Bado is suffering from influenza. Because she's dehydrated, the doctor orders I.V. therapy to replace lost body fluids. You decide to insert the line using a winged-tip needle to help reduce I.V.-associated infections. Here's how:*

Begin by gathering the necessary equipment: prescribed I.V. solution, administration set, 21G winged-tip needle (we're using a Butterfly® needle), tourniquet, 4"x4" sterile gauze pads, alcohol wipes, povidone-iodine swab, iodophor (Betadine) ointment, tape, emesis basin, and an I.V. pole.

Explain the procedure to Ms. Bado. Then, wash your hands. Remember, follow strict aseptic technique throughout this procedure.

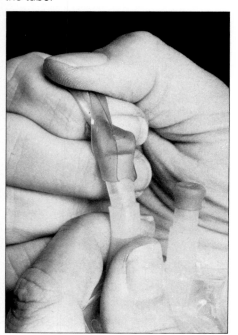

2 Now, open the package containing the I.V. solution bag. Squeeze the I.V. bag to check for leaks. If you see any, assume that the solution is contaminated. Discard the bag and obtain a replacement.

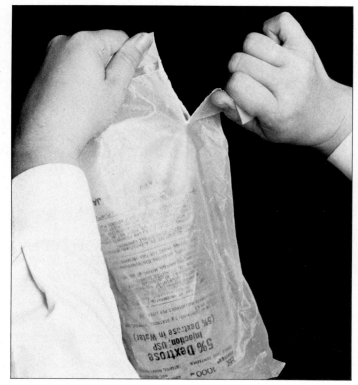

3 Now, remove the protective cap from the I.V. bag. Then, open the administration set package, maintaining aseptic technique. Close the tubing's roller clamp to prevent air from entering the tube.

4 Next, remove the spike guard and push the spike into the bag, as shown here. Be careful not to touch the outside of the bag or your hands with the spike.

Label the tubing and solution bag with the date. Hang the I.V. bag on the pole.

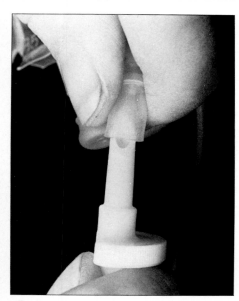

5 Next, remove the tube's protective cap and hold the exposed end over the emesis basin. Then, open the roller clamp and flush the tubing solution to expel air from the line. Doing so will prime the tubing.

Reclamp the tube, and replace the protective cap.

📖 *Nursing tip:* If the protective cap gets contaminated, cover the tube's exposed end with a capped sterile needle.

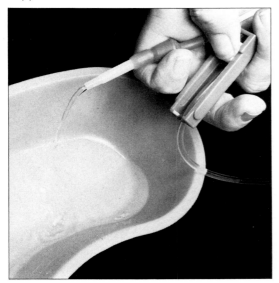

6 Now, apply a tourniquet to your patient's arm. When the tourniquet's applied properly, it will impede your patient's venous blood flow without stopping the arterial blood flow. Then, choose a vein and loosen the tourniquet.

If applying the tourniquet doesn't help you find a vein, lightly palpate the skin over the vein. Or, remove the tourniquet and apply a blood pressure cuff. Adjust the cuff pressure so it's just below Ms. Bado's systolic blood pressure.

Suppose none of these methods helps you find a vein. In this case, wrap a warm towel around your patient's arm for 10 to 20 minutes. Then, remove the towel.

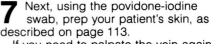

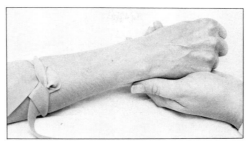

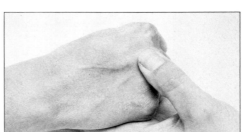

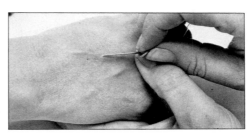

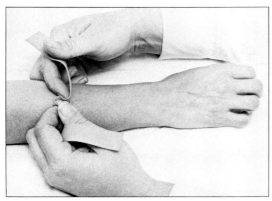

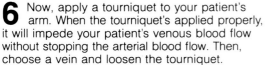

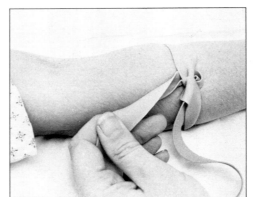

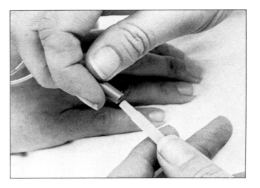

7 Next, using the povidone-iodine swab, prep your patient's skin, as described on page 113.

If you need to palpate the vein again, put on a sterile glove, or clean your fingers with an antiseptic. Next, reapply the tourniquet 1½" (3.8 cm) above the insertion site. Ask Ms. Bado to repeatedly clench and unclench her fist. Then, instruct her to keep her fist closed.

8 Hold Ms. Bado's arm securely. Then, place your thumb below the insertion site and pull her skin taut, as the nurse is doing here.

9 Now, remove the needle's protective covering. With the needle bevel up, hold the needle at a 45° angle, pointing toward the blood flow.

Insert the needle into your patient's hand.

10 Decrease the angle of the needle to 15° and direct it toward the vein. Carefully puncture the vein with the needle. Check for blood backflow in the tubing.

If you don't see any backflow, you may have missed the vein. In this case, withdraw the needle and try again with a new needle.

Release the tourniquet from your patient's arm.

11 Now, attach the I.V. tubing to the needle hub, as shown here. Then, open the roller clamp and adjust the flow rate.

Check the insertion site for signs of infiltration: warmth, redness, and swelling. If you see any, the needle may have perforated the vein's opposite wall, or not completely entered the vein. Remove the needle and insert a new one at a different site.

Percutaneous pathways

Inserting a peripheral line using a winged-tip needle continued

12 Remove the cap from the Betadine ointment. To ensure ointment sterility squeeze a small amount of ointment onto a 4"x4" sterile gauze pad and discard the pad.

Now, apply the Betadine ointment to the insertion site. Recap the ointment and put it aside.

Cover the site with an adhesive bandage.

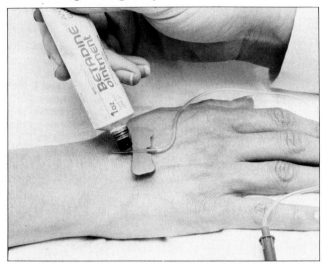

13 Now, secure the needle to your patient's hand with nonallergenic tape. To do this, place a piece of tape, sticky side up, under the needle wings. Then, cross the ends of the tape over the wings, as shown here. Place a second piece of tape over the wings, perpendicular to the needle.

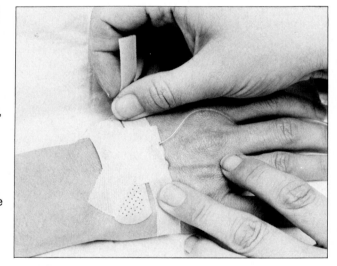

14 To prevent the needle from dislodging, loop the tubing and secure it to your patient's hand with more tape. Make sure the tape doesn't cover the connector.

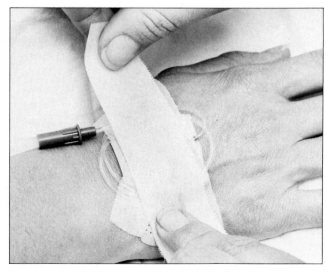

15 Next, label a piece of tape with the insertion date and time, and the needle size and type. Place it over your patient's dressing, as shown in this photo.

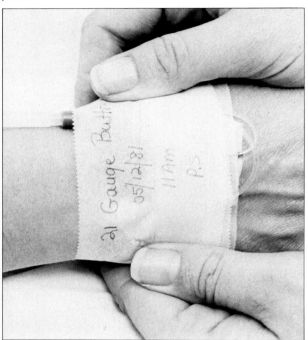

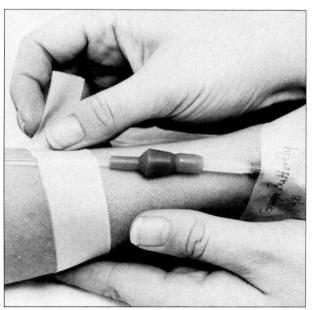

16 Tape the I.V. tubing to your patient's arm, as the nurse is doing here. This prevents the connector from being pulled, which would move the needle in your patient's vein. Remove the tourniquet.

Document the procedure in your nurses' notes, including the insertion site, time, date, needle gauge and type, flow rate, and your initials.

Inserting a peripheral I.V. line using an over-the-needle catheter (ONC)

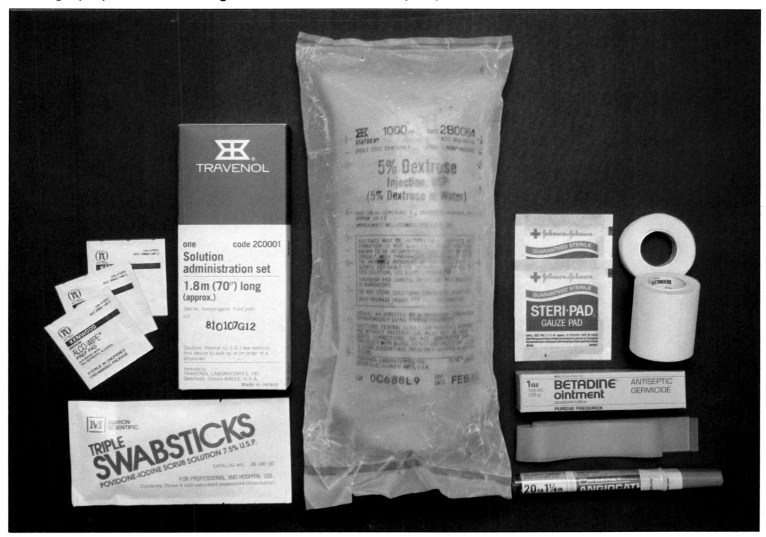

1 *Consider this: Georgeanne Swanson is scheduled for a cholecystectomy in an hour. Because the necessary I.V. line will probably remain in place only a short time, you'll insert it peripherally, using an over-the-needle catheter (ONC). Here's how:*

First, gather the necessary equipment: prescribed I.V. solution, administration set, ONC (we're using an Angiocath), tourniquet, 2"x2" sterile gauze pads, povidone-iodine (Betadine) swabs, alcohol wipes, nonallergenic tape, antimicrobial ointment, and an I.V. pole.

Explain the procedure to your patient. Then, wash your hands.

Now, prepare the site and perform venipuncture.

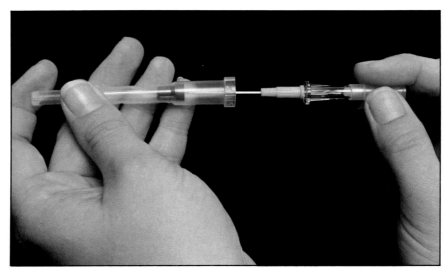

2 Remove the ONC from its protective cover, as shown here. Insert the ONC needle into your patient's vein. Holding the needle stable, advance the catheter another ¼" (0.6 cm) into the vein.

Percutaneous pathways

Inserting a peripheral I.V. line using an over-the-needle catheter (ONC) continued

3 Slip a sterile 2″x2″ gauze pad under the catheter hub when the catheter's in place. The gauze pad creates a sterile field, protecting the hub and tubing adapter from contamination.

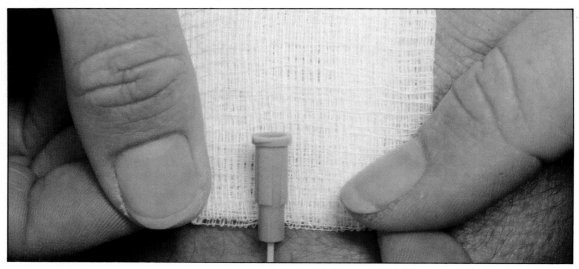

4 Carefully withdraw the needle from the catheter. If the catheter's properly placed in your patient's vein, you'll see a blood backflow in the tubing.
   What if no blood backflow appears? Then withdraw the catheter and obtain a replacement. Choose another site and begin the procedure again.

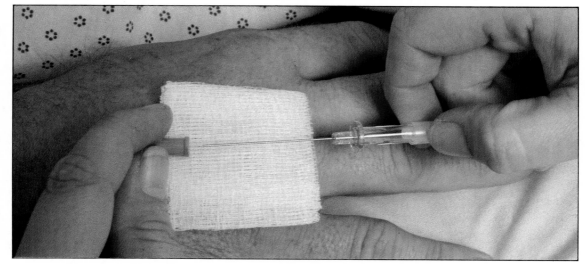

5 Now, connect the I.V. tubing to the catheter hub, as shown here.
   Open the roller clamp and set the correct flow rate. Make sure the solution's flowing freely.

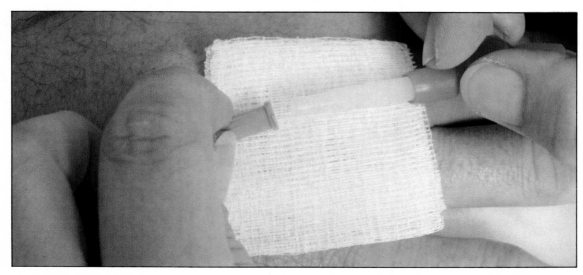

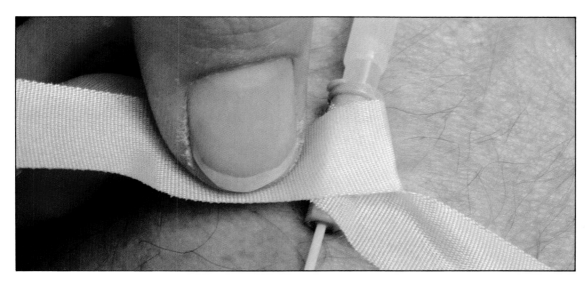

6 Place a piece of nonaller-genic tape under the catheter hub. Crisscross the tape over the hub, as shown here. Then, put a second piece of tape over the hub. To prevent contamination, avoid touching the insertion site with the tape.

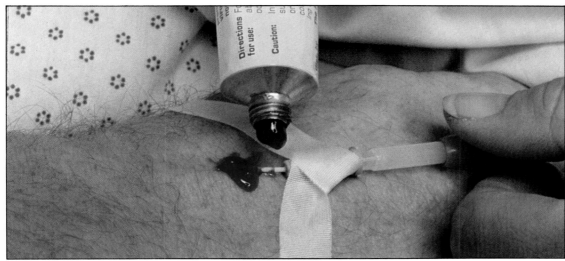

7 Apply antimicrobial oint-ment to the catheter inser-tion site, as the nurse is doing here. Cover the site with an adhesive bandage or a 2"x2" sterile gauze pad.

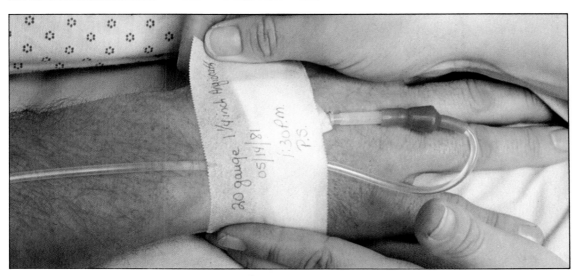

8 Loop the tubing loosely to avoid kinking, and tape it securely. Remember to mark the dressing with the insertion date and time, the needle gauge and type, and your ini-tials. Wash your hands.
  Finally, document the proce-dure in your nurses' notes.

Percutaneous pathways

Using an I.V. line filter

How does an I.V. line filter protect your patient from infection? As you know, all I.V. equipment is sterile. But contaminants can enter the I.V. line at any point. A filter may prevent some or all of these contaminants from entering your patient's bloodstream.

If your patient's receiving an I.V. admixture or a solution with special additives, using a filter becomes even more important. Why? Because these solutions may contain microorganisms and particulate matter that serve as possible sources of infection.

Filter membranes range in size from 5 microns to 0.22 microns. The finer the membrane, the more contaminants it can filter. The Ivex®2 0.22 micron filter shown below and at right may prevent even the smallest microorganisms from passing into your patient's I.V. line.

Here's how to prime and connect a filter to your patient's I.V line. Use aseptic technique throughout. Begin by closing the clamps and removing the protective cap from the drip chamber. Now, spike the I.V. bag with the filter tubing. Prime the tubing and filter by inverting the I.V. bag and squeezing the drip chamber. Then, open the clamps, running solution through the line. As the solution passes through the filter, dislodge air bubbles by inverting the filter and tapping it lightly.

When you've completed the priming procedure, remove the male adapter cover and connect the tubing to the I.V. line.

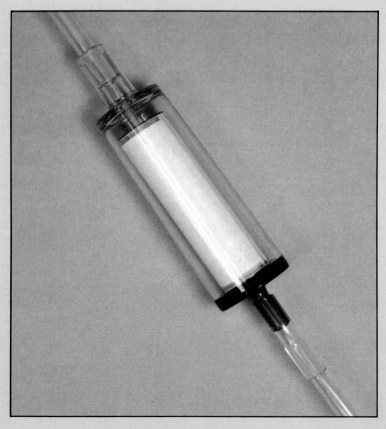

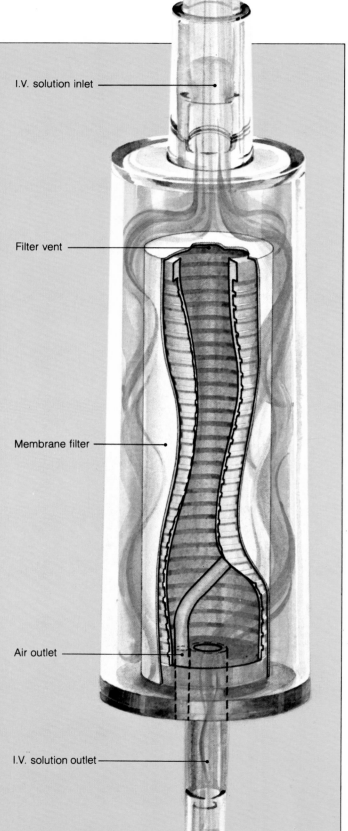

I.V. solution inlet

Filter vent

Membrane filter

Air outlet

I.V. solution outlet

Changing I.V. equipment

1 *Let's assume your patient's receiving fluid through a peripheral I.V. line. As you know, you'll need to routinely change the I.V. equipment to help prevent infection. Whenever possible, change the I.V. tubing, dressing, and solution container at the same time. By handling the equipment as little as possible, you'll minimize chances of contamination. Here's how:*

First, gather a complete set of equipment, including an I.V. administration set, several 2"x2" sterile gauze pads, a 4"x4" sterile gauze pad, antimicrobial ointment, I.V. solution, emesis basin, alcohol wipe, and nonallergenic tape.

Next, explain the procedure to your patient. Then, wash your hands thoroughly. Open the administration set, using aseptic technique.

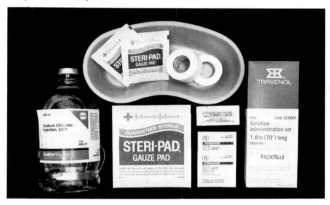

2 Now, use an alcohol wipe to clean the top of the new I.V. bag or bottle (we're using a bottle). Then, spike the bottle with the new tubing. Hang the new bottle on the pole.

Holding the exposed end of the new tubing over the emesis basin, release the clamp and flush the tubing. Make sure it doesn't touch the basin.

Then, close the roller clamp. Secure I.V. tubing by looping or taping it to the pole.

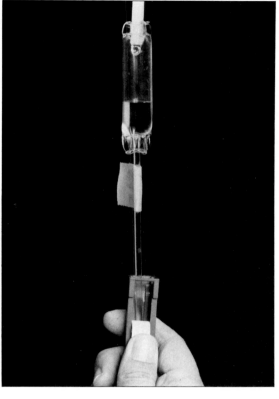

3 Next, close the roller clamp on the old tubing. Remove the old I.V. solution container from the pole and place it on a table.

Disconnect the old tubing from the container and hang or tape the tubing to the I.V. pole. Then, use the spike cover from the new tubing to cover the end of the disconnected tube. Remember, the other end of the tube is still connected to your patient.

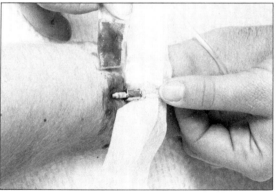

4 Hold the hub of an over-the-needle catheter (ONC) while you untape the old dressing, to avoid dislodging the catheter as you work. Tell your patient to keep his arm motionless until you've retaped the new dressing.

Discard the old dressing.

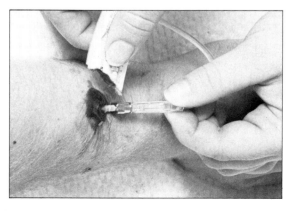

5 Clean the area around the insertion site with an alcohol wipe. Then, apply an antimicrobial ointment.

Cover the insertion site with a 2"x2" sterile gauze pad or an adhesive bandage. Secure the dressing with nonallergenic tape.

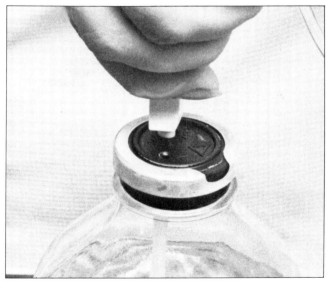

Percutaneous pathways

Changing I.V. equipment continued

6 Now, place a 4"x4" sterile gauze pad under the catheter hub to create a sterile field.

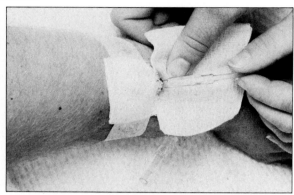

7 Remove the protective cap from the new tubing and hold the end between your fingers to keep it accessible. Then, press your finger over the catheter to hold it in place, as shown here. Grasp the hub with the gauze pad to prevent contamination.

Carefully disconnect the old tubing.

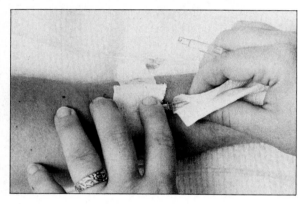

8 Next, quickly connect the new tubing to the needle hub (see photo).

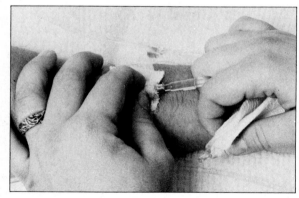

9 Now, open the roller clamp and adjust the flow rate. Use nonallergenic tape to secure the catheter to your patient's arm.

Label the dressing with the insertion time and date, and the needle gauge and type. Also, be sure to label the tubing and bottle with the date and time.

Finally, document the procedure in your nurses' notes.

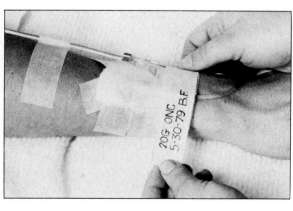

Adding a medication to an I.V. solution

1 *Let's suppose the doctor wants your patient to receive 20 mEq potassium chloride in 1,000 ml 5% dextrose in water. Because he wants the medication infused over an 8-hour period, you must administer the mixture intravenously. Here's how:*

First, gather the following equipment: potassium chloride, filter (we're using a PMF™ particulate matter filter), 12 cc syringe, two 20G 1″ needles, alcohol wipes, I.V. solution administration set, and a timing label. Make sure the equipment's sterile, the drug and dosage match the doctor's order, and the I.V. solution and medication are not outdated. Also, check the compatibility of the medication and I.V. solution.

Then, confirm your patient's identity and explain the procedure. Wash your hands.

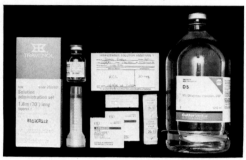

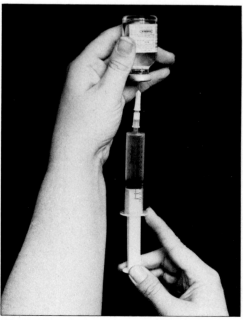

2 Now, attach the filter to the syringe. Then, connect the needle to the syringe. Clean the top of the medication vial with an alcohol wipe. Then, draw up the prescribed amount of medication into the syringe, as shown here.

3 Now, replace the filter and needle with the 20G, 1″ needle. Changing the needle prevents the medication from becoming contaminated. To minimize the risk of contamination, leave the cap on the needle.

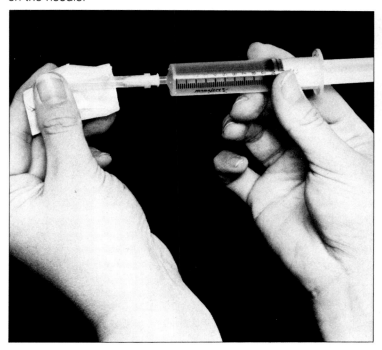

5 Uncap the needle and insert it into the port. Then, inject the medication into the solution, as shown here.

If you're transporting the I.V. bottle from another area to your patient's room, remember to cover the primary solution with a sterile additive cap.

Important: Infuse I.V. solution immediately after injecting with medication to prevent contamination.

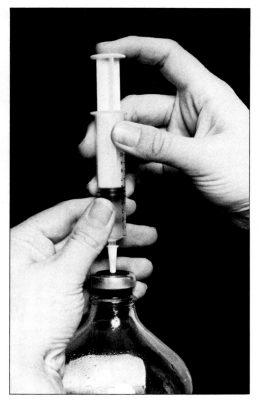

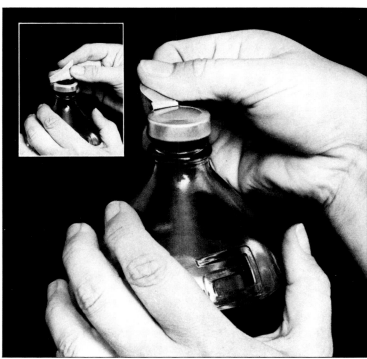

4 Next, remove the cap from the I.V. solution container. Then, clean the port with an alcohol wipe, as the nurse is doing in the inset.

6 To mix the solution, gently roll the bottle between your hands. Label the I.V. bottle, noting the added medication and strength, date, time, and your initials. Remember to affix the label upside down so it'll be easy to read when you hang the bottle.

Spike and hang the bottle on the I.V. pole. Then, start a peripheral I.V.

Document the procedure in your nurses' notes and on the medication sheet.

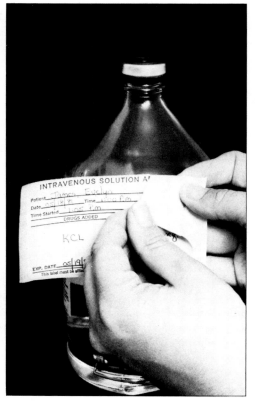

Percutaneous pathways

Administering medication: I.V. bolus

1 *Let's assume your patient, 55-year-old Donna Whitman, has a cardiac arrhythmia. The doctor orders 25 mg lidocaine hydrochloride I.V. Do you know how to safely administer medication through an I.V. line? Read this photostory to find out how.*

Note: The nurse in this story is using a Bristoject® single-dose syringe, which includes needle, syringe, and medication vial.

To begin, confirm your patient's identity and make sure the drug and dosage match the doctor's order. Next, check the medication's expiration date. Be sure the medication's compatible with your patient's I.V. solution.

Wash your hands. Then, check that the I.V. needle is placed properly in your patient's vein.

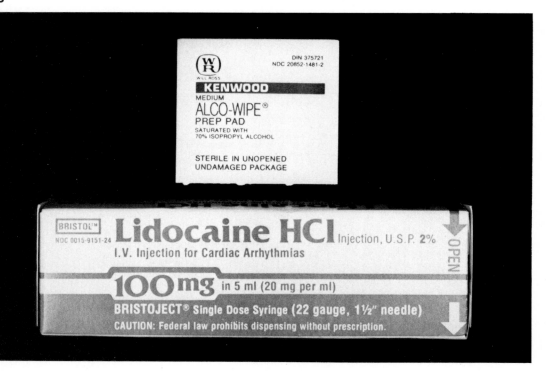

W R
WILL ROSS
DIN 375721
NDC 20852-1481-2
KENWOOD
MEDIUM
ALCO-WIPE®
PREP PAD
SATURATED WITH
70% ISOPROPYL ALCOHOL
STERILE IN UNOPENED
UNDAMAGED PACKAGE

BRISTOL™
NDC 0015-9151-24
Lidocaine HCl Injection, U.S.P. 2%
I.V. Injection for Cardiac Arrhythmias
100 mg in 5 ml (20 mg per ml)
BRISTOJECT® Single Dose Syringe (22 gauge, 1½" needle)
CAUTION: Federal law prohibits dispensing without prescription.
OPEN

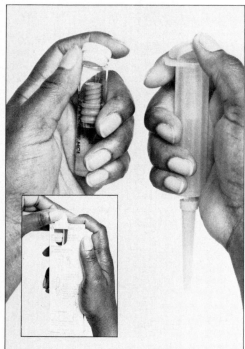

2 Now, remove the injector and vial from the package (inset). Make sure both protective caps are in place. If they're not, discard the equipment and obtain a replacement. Snap off the protective caps of the vial and injector.

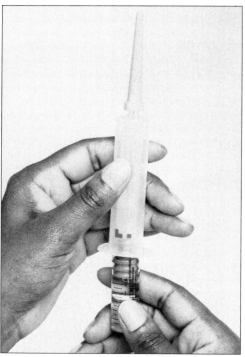

3 Holding the injector vertically, insert the vial. Then, rotate the vial clockwise three times until you feel resistance.

Continue rotating the vial about another half turn until the medication touches the needle.

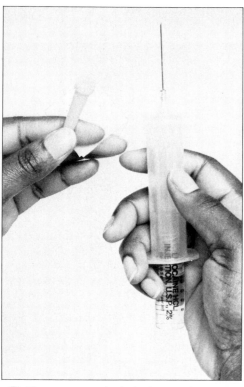

4 Now, use an alcohol wipe to clean the injection port on your patient's I.V. line. Uncap the needle and place the cap on a clean alcohol wipe.

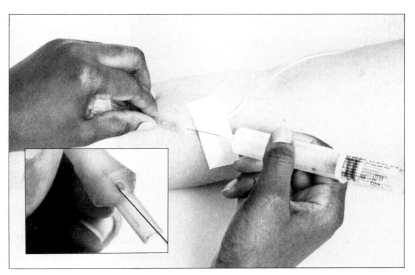

5 Hold the I.V. tubing near the port and carefully insert the needle into the injection port, as the nurse is doing here.

Does the injection port have an "O" marked on it? If so, insert the needle within this circle to prevent leakage (see inset).

Close the roller clamp.

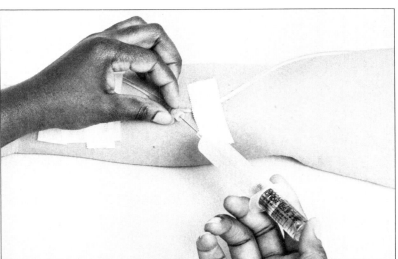

6 Next, inject the medication into the I.V. line at the prescribed rate. When you're done, remove the needle from the port and recap it.

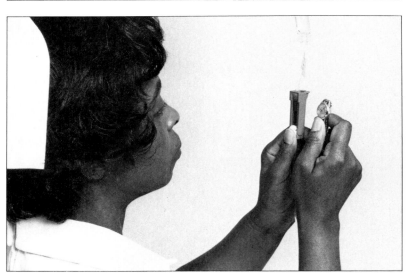

7 Now, open the roller clamp. If the medication irritates your patient's vein, let the I.V. solution flow rapidly through the tubing for about 1 minute to dilute the medication. Adjust the flow rate. Then, discard the injector, needle, and vial into the proper receptacles.

Finally, document the procedure in your nurses' notes.

Caring for a patient with a central line

Any time your patient has a central line in place, his risk of infection increases. Why? Because a central line, such as one used for central venous pressure (CVP), total parenteral nutrition (TPN), or an external cardiac pacemaker, usually remains in place longer than 48 hours. And the longer a line stays in, the greater the chance of infection.

You can reduce your patient's chance of infection by following these guidelines:
• Always maintain strict aseptic technique when caring for your patient's I.V. line or when changing his dressing.
• Change your patient's I.V. dressing every 24 hours, according to hospital policy. Always apply a sterile, air-occlusive dressing.
• Change the entire I.V. setup (including CVP manometer and transducer domes, if applicable) every 24 to 48 hours.
• Never administer medications or draw blood specimens from a central I.V. line.
• Check your patient for signs and symptoms of thrombophlebitis, such as pain or soreness in his neck, shoulder, or chest; swelling of his catheterized arm; or neck vein distention. If any occur, notify the doctor immediately.
• Notify the doctor immediately if you see any signs and symptoms of infection: redness, swelling, oozing pus at the catheter site, or sudden development of a fever. He may want you to remove the catheter and culture the tip (see page 27 for details) or obtain blood cultures.
• Does your patient have a CVP line? Don't let the filter at the top of the manometer get wet. If it does, change it immediately.
• If your patient has a Swan-Ganz catheter in place, never allow blood to back up into the transducer lines.

Percutaneous pathways

Inserting a central I.V. line: Your role

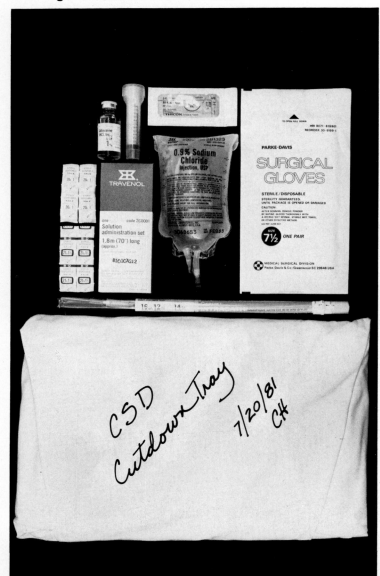

1 *Consider this situation: The doctor orders total parenteral nutrition (TPN) for 48-year-old Mary Carson. He'll be inserting a central I.V. line through your patient's subclavian vein and wants you to assist. Do you know how? If you're unsure, read this story.*

First, gather the necessary equipment: venisection tray (cutdown tray), 3-0 silk with Keith needle, 16G 12" catheter, gloves, normal saline solution, sterile water, administration tubing, 10 cc syringe, assorted needles, anesthetic, povidone-iodine solution swabsticks, antimicrobial ointment, 4"x4" and 2"x2" sterile gauze pads, and two gauze masks (optional according to hospital policy). You'll also need nonallergenic tape, soap, an emesis basin, a folded sheet, and an I.V. pole.

Explain the procedure to Ms. Carson and reassure her. Then, wash your hands with an antiseptic.

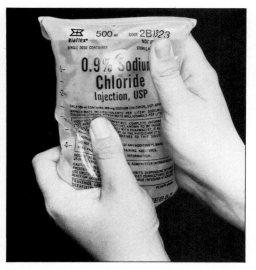

2 Examine the normal saline solution container (here we're using a bag). If you see any leaks or solution inconsistency (such as cloudiness or precipitate), discard the bag and obtain a replacement.

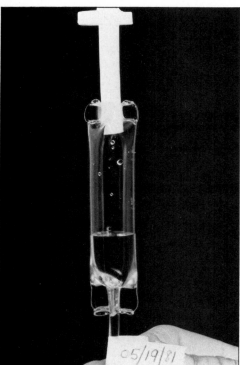

3 If everything's okay, insert the administration tubing into the solution bag, using aseptic technique. Invert the bag and hang it on the I.V. pole. Mark the date on the tubing and solution bag.

Next, remove the tube's protective cap and point the exposed end into an emesis basin. Flush the tubing with the solution and replace the protective cap.

4 Now, position your patient flat on her back. Be sure to remove the pillow from the bed. Remove your patient's gown from her shoulders. Clean the subclavian area with soap and sterile water. Then, cover her shoulders with a drape until the procedure begins.

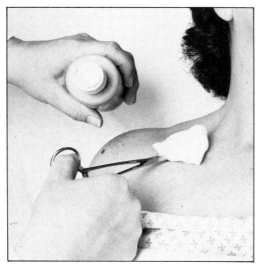

5 Roll the folded sheet and place it between your patient's shoulder blades, as shown here. This position will hyperextend her shoulders, encouraging vein distention.

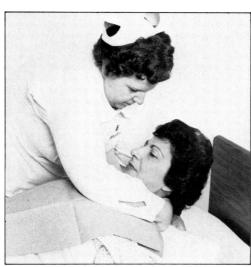

6 Then, adjust her bed to the Trendelenburg position to increase the venous pressure in your patient's upper thorax and reduce the risk of an air embolism.
 Remove the drape from your patient's shoulders, and turn her head away from the site.

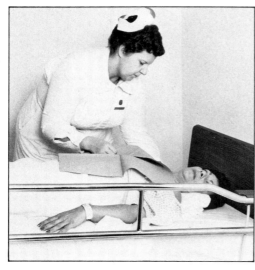

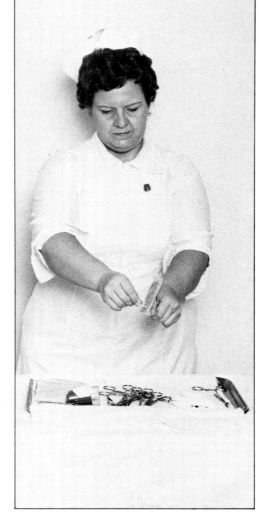

7 Maintaining aseptic technique, unwrap the sterile gloves and 4"x4" gauze pads, and open the venipuncture tray. Then, open the suture material and catheter package, being careful not to do this directly over the sterile field. Drop the sutures and catheter into the opened sterile tray.

8 Now, the doctor will scrub the insertion site with the povidone-iodine solution swabsticks. Then, he'll put on sterile gloves and drape your patient's shoulder with sterile towels, leaving only a small area exposed.

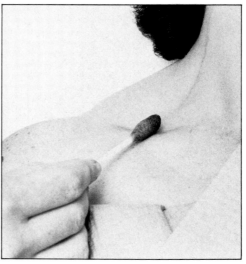

Percutaneous pathways

Inserting a central I.V. line: Your role continued

9 Next, the doctor will inject a local anesthetic at the insertion site.

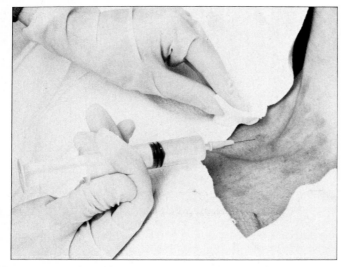

10 Then, he'll insert the catheter needle into the patient's subclavian vein.
  Throughout the procedure, continue to reassure your patient and monitor heart rhythm closely.

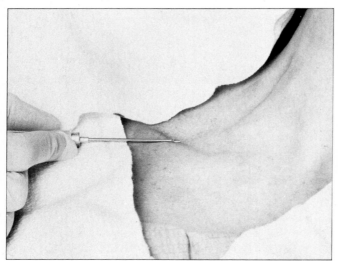

11 Next, connect the solution tubing to the catheter, as shown here. Open the roller clamp and adjust the flow rate.
  Then, momentarily lower the bag below the level of the insertion site to check for blood return in the tubing. This ensures patency and proper placement.

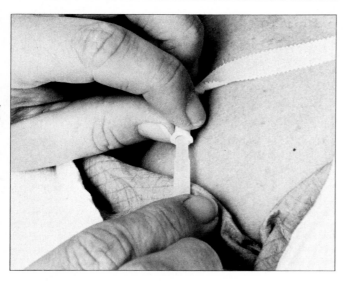

12 Once the doctor's sutured and taped the catheter to your patient's skin, apply antimicrobial ointment to the insertion site.

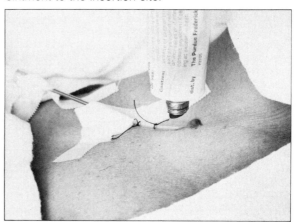

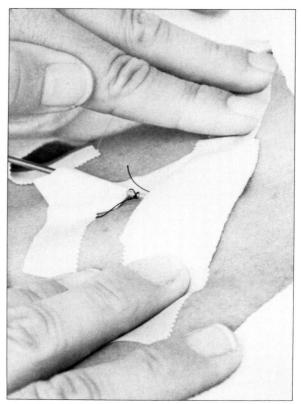

13 Cover the site with a 2"x2" sterile gauze pad. Secure the gauze pad with nonallergenic tape, forming a temporary dressing.
  When catheter placement has been confirmed by X-ray, apply the air-occlusive dressing.
  Mark the insertion time, date, and the doctor's initials on the tape. Document the catheter size, site and solution flow rate in your nurses' notes. Also, make a note that the catheter placement was confirmed by X-ray.

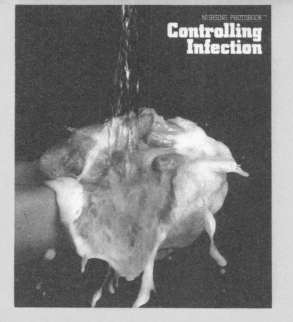

NURSING PHOTOBOOK™
Controlling Infection

10-DAY FREE TRIAL

USE THESE CARDS TO:

1. **Join the NURSING PHOTOBOOK™ series, with *Controlling Infection* as your first volume. $12.95 per book.**

    or

2. **Buy extra copies of *Controlling Infection* without joining the series. $14.95 per book.**

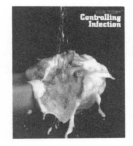

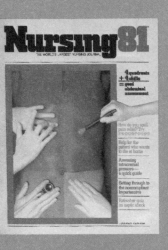

GET ACQUAINTED WITH THE WORLD'S LARGEST NURSING JOURNAL TODAY!

Mail the postage-paid card at right. ▶

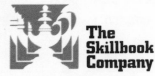
Controlling Infection…your
introduction to the brand-new NURSING PHOTOBOOK™ series.

…the remarkable breakthrough in nursing education that can change your career. Each book in this unique series contains detailed *Photostories*… and tables, charts, and graphs to help you learn important new procedures. And each handsome Photobook offers you
• 160 illustrated, fact-filled pages • brilliant, high-contrast photographs • convenient 9″ × 10½″ size • durable, hardcover binding • carefully chosen bibliography • complete index. Watch the experts at work showing you how to… administer drugs… teach your patient about his illness and its treatment… minimize trauma… understand doctors' diagnoses… increase patient comfort… and much more. Discover how you can become a better nurse by joining this exciting series.

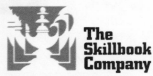
10-DAY FREE TRIAL

USE THESE CARDS TO:

1. **Join the NURSING PHOTOBOOK™ series, with *Controlling Infection* as your first volume. $12.95 per book.**

   or

2. **Buy extra copies of *Controlling Infection* without joining the series. $14.95 per book.**

© 1981 Intermed Communications. Inc.

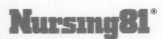
Be sure to mail the postage-paid card at left to reserve *your* first copy of *Nursing81*.

Nursing81 gives you clear, concise instruction in "hands-on" nursing. Every issue brings you in-depth clinical articles about the newest developments in nursing care—what's being discovered, researched, treated, cured. You'll learn about the new procedures, new techniques, new medications, and new equipment that will mean more skills and knowledge for you… better care for your patients!

Order *your* subscription today!

Changing the tubing on a central line

1 *Whenever you care for a patient with a central line, you'll need to change the I.V. tubing every 24 hours. Here's how:*

Note: To minimize infection, change your patient's tubing when replacing his I.V. solution container.

Maintaining aseptic technique, remove the tubing from its package and prime it.

Then, explain the procedure to your patient. Tell him how to perform Valsalva's maneuver. (This maneuver creates internal pressure and makes an air embolism less likely.)

Important: Valsalva's maneuver is contraindicated for a patient with a cardiac disorder.

Place your patient flat on his back. Then, wash your hands thoroughly and put on sterile gloves.

Place a 2"x2" sterile gauze pad under the catheter connection, creating a sterile field.

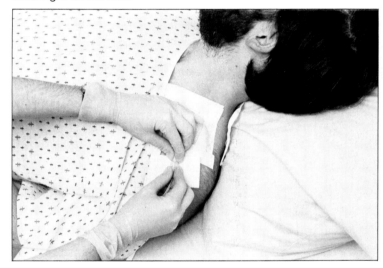

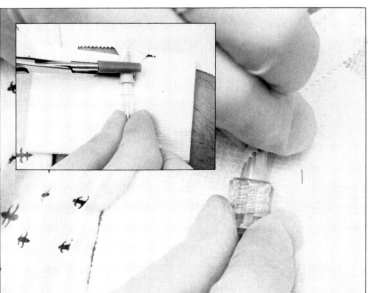

2 Now, unscrew the Luer connection (if there is one).
[Inset] Then, use a hemostat to keep the hub of the catheter steady as you disconnect the tubing.

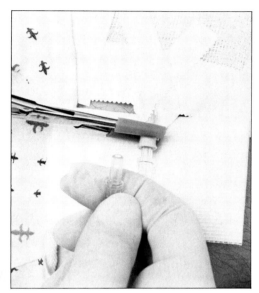

3 Next, as your patient performs Valsalva's maneuver, twist the used tubing until it detaches from the hub. Now, quickly insert the new primed tubing.

Screw the Luer connection onto the catheter hub.

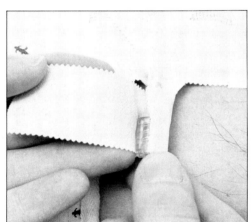

4 Next, tape the connection, as shown here. Make sure it's secure.

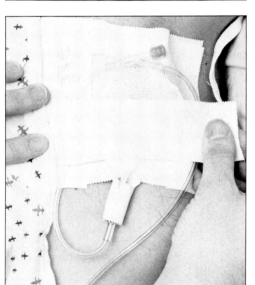

5 Loop the tubing on top of the dressing and tape it. Doing so prevents the tubing from being accidentally dislodged.

Encourage your patient to relax during therapy.

Discard the used tubing. Wash your hands. Then, document the entire procedure in your nurses' notes. Remember to label the new tubing, including when it must be changed.

Percutaneous pathways

Changing the dressing: Central line

1 *Caring for a patient with a central I.V. line? If so, you'll need to change her dressing every 24 to 48 hours, according to your hospital's policy. But, if the dressing becomes wet or loose, change it immediately. Read this photostory to learn how.*

First, gather the following equipment: disposal bag for soiled dressing; nonsterile and sterile gloves; 4″x4″ sterile gauze pads; 2″x2″ sterile precut gauze pads (we're using Sof-Wick® I.V. sponges);

povidone-iodine solution swabsticks; tincture of benzoin; antimicrobial ointment, such as Betadine; acetone; nonallergenic tape (½″ and 2″ wide), and face masks for you and your patient (as needed, following hospital policy).

Note: Keep a tray with individual dressing supplies in each patient's room. Make sure the tray remains covered when not in use.

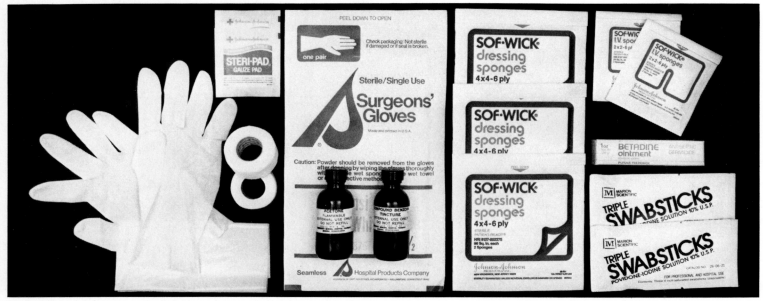

2 Now, wash your hands thoroughly and put on your face mask. Explain the procedure to your patient. Tell her she can help reduce the chance of infection by putting on a face mask and turning her head to one side. Then, help her into a supine position.

Important: Never place a mask on a patient who needs oxygen or who has a nasogastric tube in place.

Then, open your sterile supplies. Remember, you'll follow aseptic technique during the entire procedure.

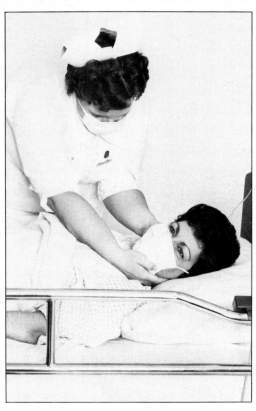

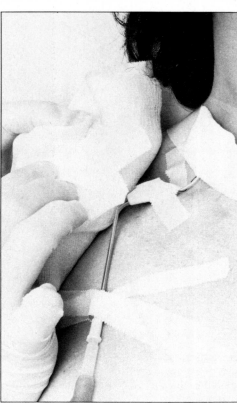

3 Now, put on the nonsterile gloves and remove the old dressing, as shown here. Take care not to disturb the catheter. Fold the soiled surfaces of the dressing together. Then, discard the dressing and gloves in the disposal bag.

4 Inspect the insertion site for signs of infection, such as purulent discharge and inflammation. If you see any, obtain a drainage specimen for culture (as described on pages 44 to 47), and send it to the lab. Then, notify the doctor.

Make sure the catheter's positioned correctly and the sutures are intact. If the catheter's taped in place, remove the soiled tape.

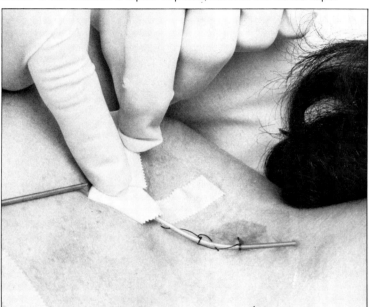

5 Next, wash your hands and put on the sterile gloves. Using a 4"x4" gauze pad soaked in acetone, clean the area around the insertion site. Use a circular motion, working from the site outward.

Note: If your patient has sensitive skin, clean the area more gently. Vigorous rubbing may cause a skin abrasion.

Be careful not to touch the catheter with the acetone-soaked gauze pad. Doing so may corrode it.

Suppose you do get acetone on the catheter. Then, wipe the catheter immediately with sterile, normal saline solution.

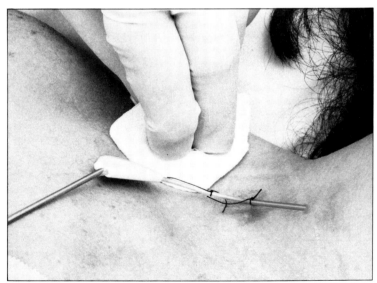

6 Clean the area surrounding the insertion site using povidone-iodine solution swabs. Then, apply Betadine ointment directly at the insertion site. Using a sterile swab, apply tincture of benzoin. Let it dry for about 1 minute.

Fit the precut sponges around the catheter so the slits overlap (see inset).

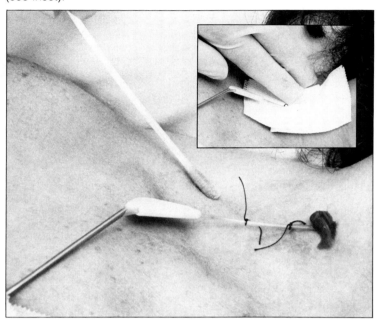

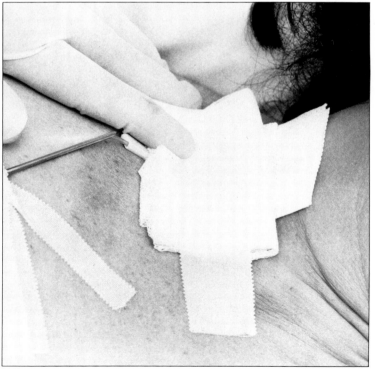

7 Fold a 4"x4" sterile gauze pad in half. Place it over the insertion site. Secure the dressing on all sides with nonallergenic tape.

Percutaneous pathways

Changing the dressing: Central line continued

8 Now, to make the dressing air-occlusive, cover it completely with nonallergenic tape, as shown here. Make sure the tape covers the catheter, but not the connection hub.

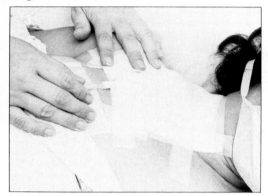

9 Now, use ½" (1.3 cm) wide adhesive tape to secure the catheter-tubing junction. To do this properly, cross under and over the junction with the tape, as shown. Apply a second piece of tape to keep the junction from separating.

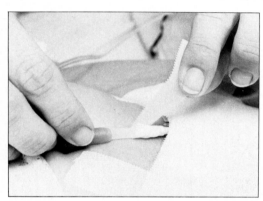

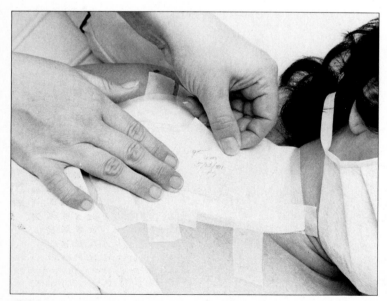

10 Next, apply a layer of nonallergenic tape to further secure the dressing.

Label the dressing with the time, date, and your initials. Seal the plastic bag containing the soiled dressing and remove the bag from your patient's room. Discard it, according to hospital policy.

Finally, wash your hands thoroughly. Then, document the procedure in your nurses' notes, including the condition of the insertion site and any specimens taken for culture.

Removing the central I.V. line

1 *Now, the doctor has ordered Ms. Carson's central I.V. line removed. If this is a nursing responsibility in your hospital, follow these steps:*

Note: If the doctor suspects an infection, he may want you to send the catheter tip to the lab for culture (see page 27 for details).

Begin by gathering the following equipment: 4"x4" sterile gauze pads, nonallergenic tape, acetone, sterile gloves, adhesive bandage strip, antimicrobial ointment, povidone-iodine solution (such as Betadine), and a sterile instrument set (containing forceps and scissors).

Explain the procedure to your patient. Place her in a supine position and expose her dressing.

Then, wash your hands.

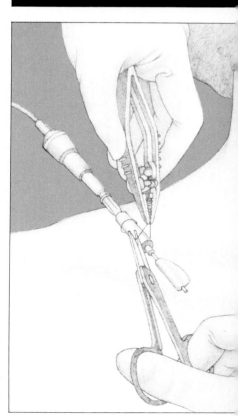

2 Now, carefully loosen the tape on the dressing. As you remove the dressing, fold the soiled sides together.

🖐 *Nursing tip:* Wear gloves to protect your hands from contamination.

Next, inspect the insertion site for signs of infection, such as purulent drainage. If you see any, culture the wound drainage and send it to the lab. Be sure your wound culture specimen doesn't include contaminants from the skin.

Wash your hands and put on the sterile gloves. Use the sterile scissors to remove the sutures securing the catheter.

Important: Make sure you don't cut through the catheter when removing the sutures.

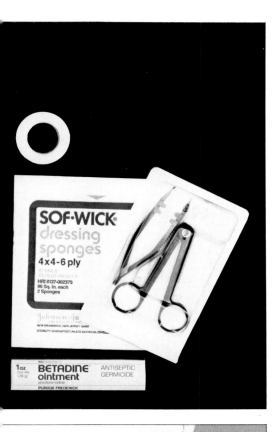

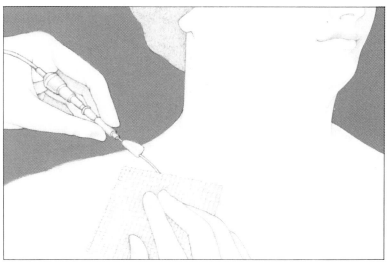

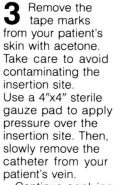

3 Remove the tape marks from your patient's skin with acetone. Take care to avoid contaminating the insertion site. Use a 4″x4″ sterile gauze pad to apply pressure over the insertion site. Then, slowly remove the catheter from your patient's vein.

Continue applying pressure for 1 minute after the catheter's removed.

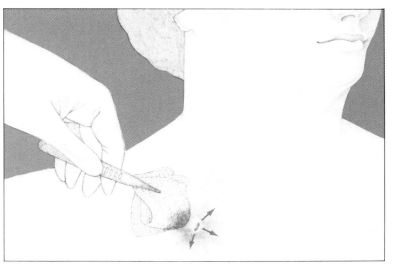

4 Clean the area with povidone-iodine solution. Then, apply antimicrobial ointment to the insertion site. Cover the site with a pressure bandage. Secure with tape.

After 1 hour, you'll need to remove the bandage, apply additional antimicrobial ointment, and cover the site with an adhesive bandage strip.

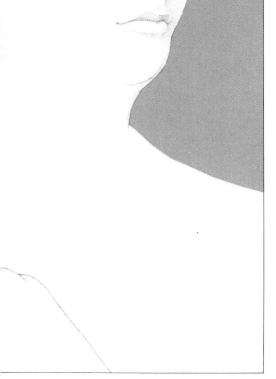

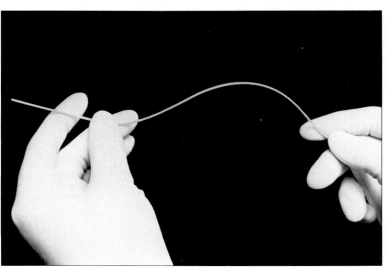

5 Now, examine the catheter closely. If the tip is ragged or damaged, suspect a catheter embolism. Notify the doctor.

Remove the gloves and wash your hands. Document in your notes the date, time, and insertion site and catheter condition. Also include the dressing and ointment applied, and any culturing information if applicable.

Percutaneous pathways

Assisting with thoracentesis

1 *Picture this: Dan Brager, a 28-year-old hairdresser, has been admitted to your unit with dyspnea and chest pains. The doctor suspects pleural effusion and decides to perform a thoracentesis. She asks you to assist. Here's how:*

First, gather the following equipment: sterile gloves, and a thoracentesis tray containing: three-way stopcock; 5 cc Stylex® syringe; 5 ml lidocaine hydrochloride; 25G ⅜" needle; 22G 2" needle; three prenumbered specimen tubes with caps; two swabsticks; puncture site bandage; sterile towel and drapes. You'll also need povidone-

iodine solution.

If the doctor'll be doing a biopsy, she'll also need a biopsy needle and a sterile container of formalin.

Note: Some doctors attach a hemostat to the needle. That way, the needle won't accidentally penetrate too deeply and injure the patient's lung.

Then, thoroughly explain the procedure to Mr. Brager. Be sure to answer any questions he may have. Tell him he may feel some pain when the needle's inserted. Remind him not to move or cough while the needle's in his chest cavity.

3 What if your patient has trouble remaining in this position? Then, have him lie down on his unaffected side, close to the edge of the bed. Instruct him to place his arm over his head to help separate his ribs and allow easier insertion.

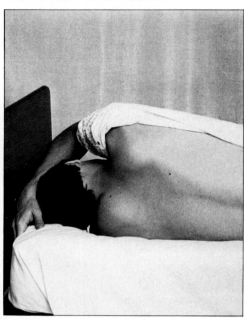

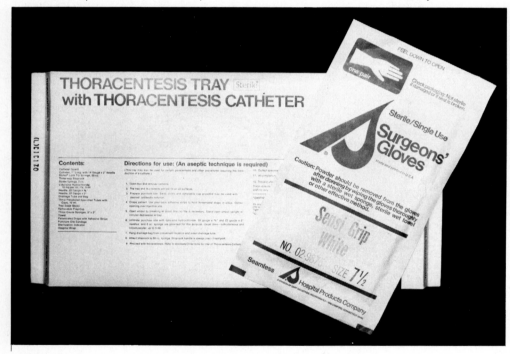

2 Position the patient sitting up with his arms supported by the overbed table, or as ordered (see photo).

Depending on the doctor's preference, you may also position the patient sitting up straight at the edge of the bed with his hand on the opposite shoulder (see inset).

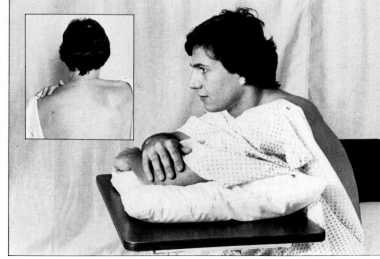

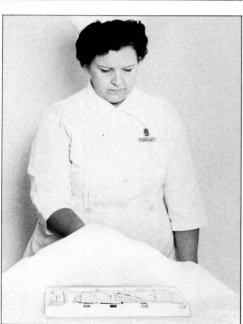

4 To create a sterile field, unwrap the thoracentesis tray, as the nurse is doing here. Be careful not to touch the tray's inner contents with your hands. If you do, you'll need to discard the tray and get a new one.

5 Now, open the package with the sterile gloves. The doctor will remove the inner package and put on the gloves.

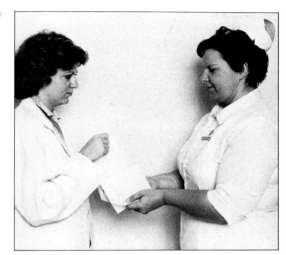

6 At this point, the doctor will be cleaning around the insertion site with gauze pads moistened with povidone-iodine solution. Then, she'll drape the area with sterile towels.

Using a 5 cc syringe, the doctor will draw up the anesthetic and inject it at the insertion site. (This will create a skin wheal.)

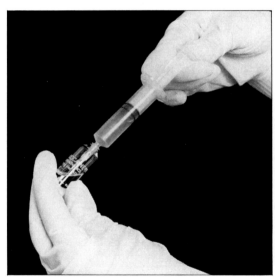

7 With a larger needle, she'll anesthetize the intercostal muscles (see illustration).

Once the needle's penetrated into your patient's outer pleura, the doctor will begin aspirating fluid into the syringe. To do this, she'll use a 50 cc syringe with a 3" large-bore needle and three-way stopcock.

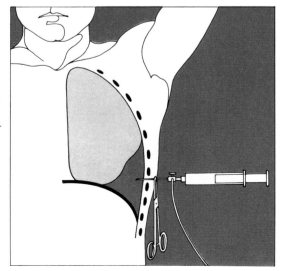

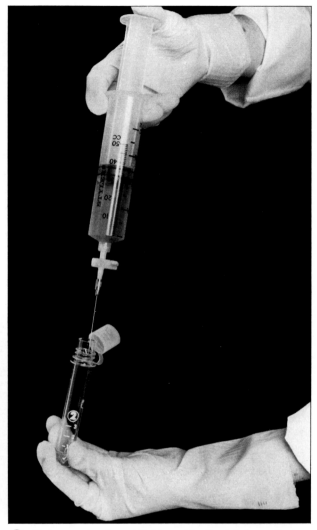

8 If she wants pleural fluid sent to the lab for culturing, she'll fill three sterile tubes. After capping each tube, she'll hand it to you. You'll need to number each tube sequentially with a grease pencil (unless the tubes are prenumbered).

Does the doctor want a biopsy specimen? If so, hold the open sterile container while the doctor places the tissue specimen inside. Carefully put on the lid, making sure you don't contaminate the inside of the lid or the container.

When the procedure's completed, help Mr. Brager into a more comfortable position. Apply a dressing over the puncture site.

Immediately thereafter, send the collected specimens to the lab with appropriate lab slips. Discard the disposable items into the appropriate receptacle. Clean all reusable items and return them to the central supply department for sterilization and recycling. Wash your hands.

Document the procedure and your patient's vital signs in your nurses' notes.

Surgical wounds

Carrie Jones just returned to your unit after having an appendectomy. Besides pulmonary complications and hemorrhage, do you know what other complications threaten Carrie's complete recovery? Surgical wound infection, for one. Do you know how to prevent this type of infection? For example, do you know how to create a sterile field? Or protect the field from contamination? Do you know how to change your patient's dressing using aseptic technique? Or prevent cross contamination from dressing supplies?

And what about the patient with a burn? Can you provide emergency care while maintaining aseptic technique? Or protect your patient from infection while using hydrotherapy equipment?

On the following pages, you'll find the answers to these questions as well as additional information to sharpen your nursing skills.

Preventing infection

Your responsibility in preventing and controlling infection at a surgical site begins before surgery, and ends when the wound healing's complete. And, if your patient has a draining wound, your responsibility increases. Why? Because, unlike a closed wound, a draining wound stays open longer, allowing microorganisms to enter the body.

How can you help prevent a surgical site infection? For starters, always wash your hands before and after each patient contact, and maintain strict aseptic technique throughout every procedure. And, before surgery, teach your patient how to properly care for his surgical wound.

Tell your patient that he may be asked to bathe with skin antiseptic before going to the operating room. Also, inform him that the surgical site will be shaved as near to the time of surgery as possible, following hospital policy. Shaving too early allows microorganisms to colonize in skin nicks or hair follicles.

Note: Does your hospital dictate usage of a depilatory to remove hair? If so, patch test a small area of your patient's skin for sensitivity.

After surgery, use only wound care supplies that are sterile. Check each supply package for tears or punctures before using it. To help prevent cross contamination, store individual dressings, antimicrobial ointments, and cleaning agents in your patient's room.

Most likely, your patient will need some type of invasive therapy after surgery; for example, an I.V. line or Foley catheter. Make sure the I.V. line or tube (if applicable) is properly dated, taped, and changed. To reduce infection risk, remove the I.V. line or tube as ordered, as soon as your patient's condition stabilizes.

Every time you change your patient's dressing, examine his wound closely for signs of infection: warmth, redness, swelling, unpleasant odor, or purulent drainage. If you note any of these signs, call the doctor immediately. He may want a drainage specimen cultured and sent to the lab. To prevent the infection from spreading, be ready to initiate wound and skin precautions, as needed.

Finally, when your patient's ready to be discharged, explain how to care for his wound at home. Show him how to properly change the dressing and apply the appropriate wound ointment, if necessary. Tell him to call the doctor immediately if he notes any of the signs of wound infection. Remember, always document everything in your nurses' notes.

Creating a sterile field: Some tips

Creating a sterile field is always your first step in any procedure requiring aseptic technique. Why? Because a sterile field helps protect your patient from contamination.

How can you create a sterile field? One way is to place a sterile towel on a flat surface; for example, a bedside table. Then, be careful not to touch that part of the towel. Using aseptic technique, open the supplies.

Important: Never open the supplies over your sterile field. Instead, use sterile forceps to transfer the sterile supplies from their wrappers to the towel. Or, after opening the wrappers outside the sterile field, carefully drop the supplies directly onto the towel.

Does the aseptic procedure you're performing require sterile solution? If so, pour the solution into a sterile basin, without touching the solution container to the basin. Avoid splashing the solution onto the sterile field.

And remember, *never* reach across your sterile field during the procedure. Doing so contaminates the supplies.

Redressing a closed wound

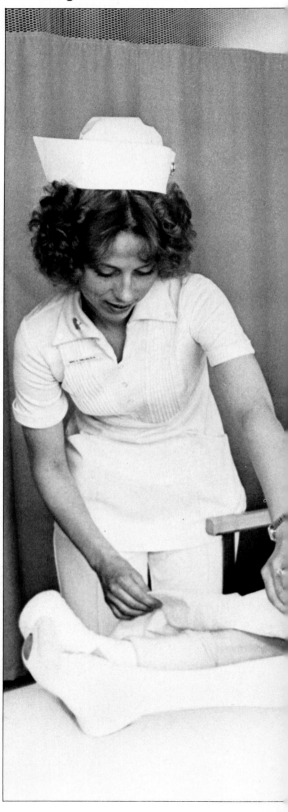

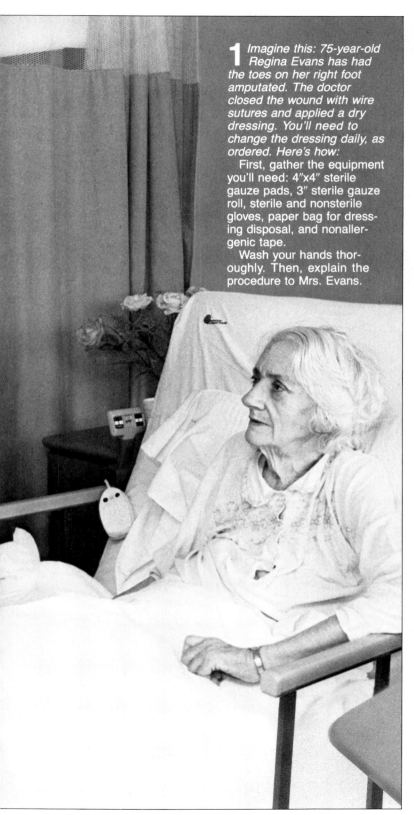

1 *Imagine this: 75-year-old Regina Evans has had the toes on her right foot amputated. The doctor closed the wound with wire sutures and applied a dry dressing. You'll need to change the dressing daily, as ordered. Here's how:*

First, gather the equipment you'll need: 4"x4" sterile gauze pads, 3" sterile gauze roll, sterile and nonsterile gloves, paper bag for dressing disposal, and nonallergenic tape.

Wash your hands thoroughly. Then, explain the procedure to Mrs. Evans.

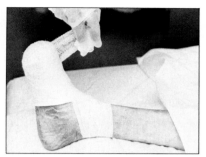

2 Put on your nonsterile gloves.
Then, unwrap the gauze that covers Mrs. Evans' dressing, as shown here.

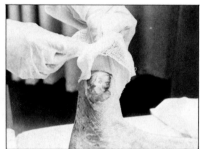

3 Carefully remove the soiled dressing from Mrs. Evans' foot. Discard the soiled dressing in the bag. Then, remove your gloves and discard them in the bag. Wash your hands.

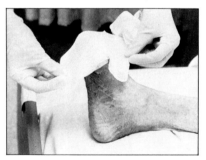

4 Using aseptic technique, open your sterile supplies. Then, put on the sterile gloves. Now, apply a 4"x4" sterile gauze pad over Mrs. Evans' wound, as the nurse is doing here.

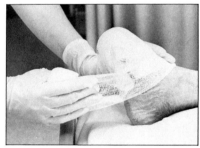

5 To secure the gauze pad, wrap the roll of gauze over the pad and around Mrs. Evans' foot.

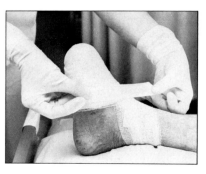

6 Tape the gauze in place, as shown here.
Finally, remove your gloves and discard them into the paper bag. Then, close the bag and place it in the appropriate covered trash receptacle. Wash your hands thoroughly.

Document the procedure, including wound appearance, in your nurses' notes.

Surgical wounds

Redressing an open wound

1 *Consider this: 35-year-old Dennis Thompson has an infection on his right arm. After the doctor performs an incision and drainage (I and D) procedure, he orders Mr. Thompson's dressing changed four times a day in preparation for a skin graft. Meanwhile, Mr. Thompson's transferred to isolation. Do you know how to change the dressing using strict aseptic technique? If you're unsure, read this story.*

First, gather the equipment: 4"x4" sterile gauze pads, povidone-iodine (Betadine) solution, 3" wide sterile gauze roll, sterile and nonsterile gloves, nonallergenic tape, paper bag for dressing disposal, and sterile Surgipads™.

Because Mr. Thompson was placed in isolation, put on an isolation gown before entering his room.

Now, explain the procedure to Mr. Thompson and expose his dressing.

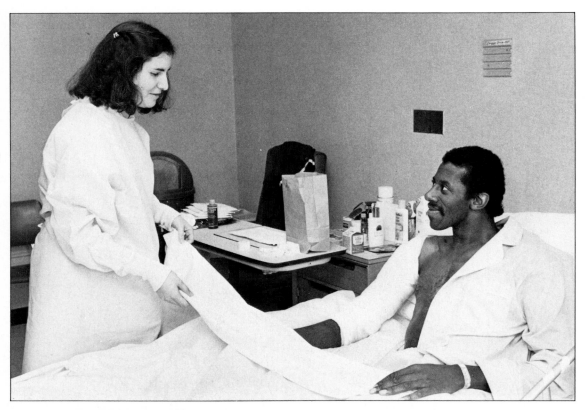

2 Wash your hands. Now, open all your sterile supplies, creating a sterile field. Squeeze the Betadine solution over the 4"x4" sterile gauze pads until they're completely saturated. Then, put on the nonsterile disposable gloves.

Carefully remove the gauze covering Mr. Thompson's soiled dressing.

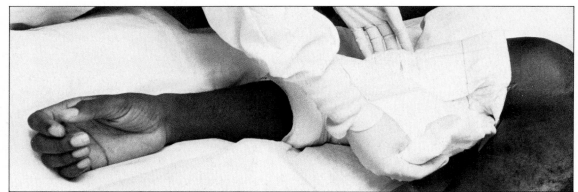

3 Next, remove the soiled dressing from his arm. Fold the dressing—contaminated sides in—as shown here. Remember, don't touch the open wound with your gloves.

Discard the dressing in the paper bag (see inset). Then, remove your gloves and discard them in the bag. Close the paper bag immediately to prevent the microorganisms from becoming airborne.

Wash your hands thoroughly.

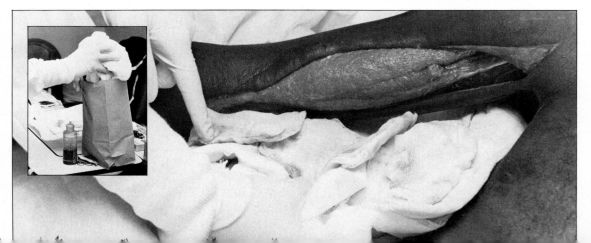

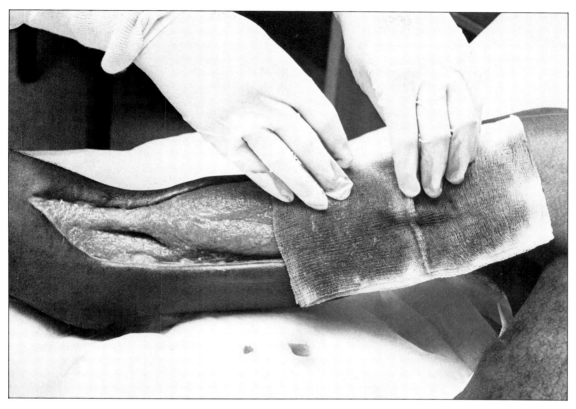

4 Now, put on your sterile gloves. Using aseptic technique, apply the saturated 4"x4" sterile gauze pads over the open wound, as the nurse is doing here. Make sure the gauze pads completely cover the wound.

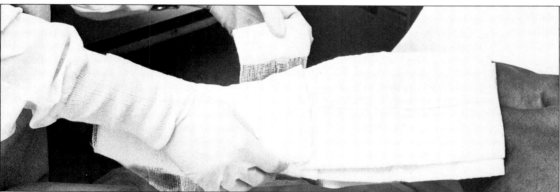

5 Next, cover the 4"x4" gauze pads with new Surgipads. To secure the dressing in place, wrap the roll of gauze around the dressing, as shown here.
Then, tape down the open end of the gauze.
Important: To prevent skin irritation, keep the tape from touching the patient's skin.

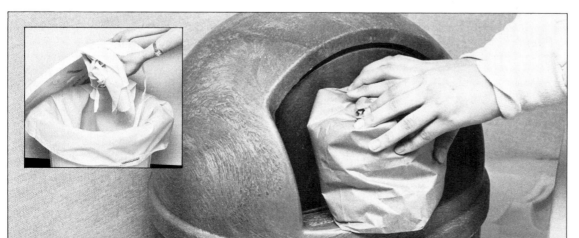

6 Now, remove your sterile gloves and discard them and the closed paper bag in the covered trash receptacle.
[Inset]Remove your isolation garb and place the items in the proper receptacles. Then, wash your hands thoroughly.
Document the procedure in your nurses' notes. Be sure to include wound appearance and any drainage or unpleasant odor.

Surgical wounds

**Caring for a patient
with a surgical wound and drain**

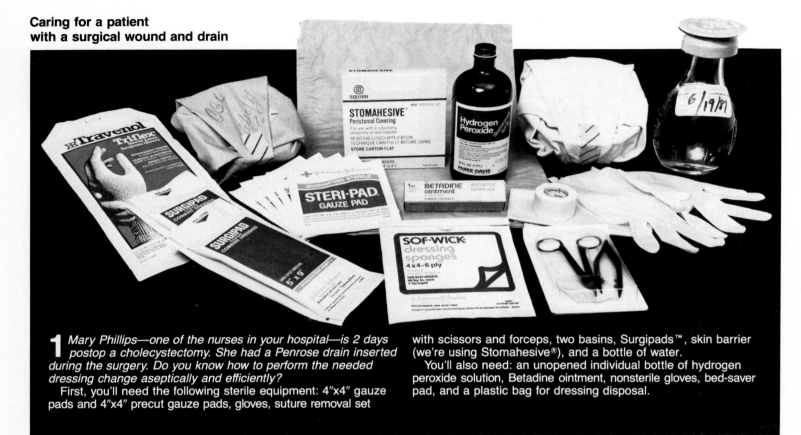

1 *Mary Phillips—one of the nurses in your hospital—is 2 days postop a cholecystectomy. She had a Penrose drain inserted during the surgery. Do you know how to perform the needed dressing change aseptically and efficiently?*

First, you'll need the following sterile equipment: 4"x4" gauze pads and 4"x4" precut gauze pads, gloves, suture removal set with scissors and forceps, two basins, Surgipads™, skin barrier (we're using Stomahesive®), and a bottle of water.

You'll also need: an unopened individual bottle of hydrogen peroxide solution, Betadine ointment, nonsterile gloves, bed-saver pad, and a plastic bag for dressing disposal.

2 Then, wash your hands and dry them with a paper towel. Now, explain the procedure to your patient. Expose her dressing, but provide a drape to keep her warm. Place a bed-saver pad under her right side. Put the opened plastic bag on the bed next to your patient.

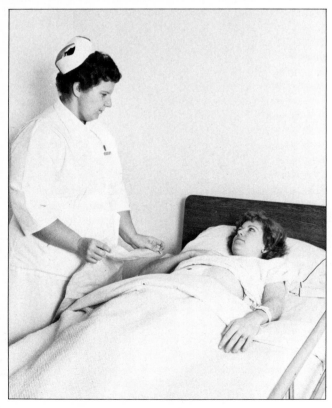

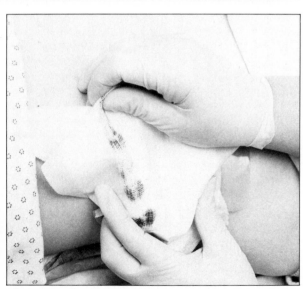

3 Now, loosen the tape around your patient's dressing. Put on the nonsterile gloves and gently remove the soiled dressing. Take care not to dislodge your patient's Penrose drain.

Fold the soiled sides of the dressing together so they don't contaminate your gloves. Place the dressing in the plastic bag. Remove your gloves and discard them in the plastic bag.

Wash your hands.

4 Maintaining sterility, open the packages of sterile 4″x4″ gauze pads. Leaving the pads in their open wrappers, place them on the bedside table. Follow this procedure with the Stomahesive, Surgipads, and suture removal set.

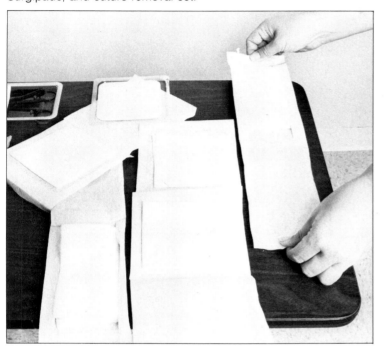

5 Still maintaining sterility, remove the wrappers from both basins, as shown here. Place the basins on the bedside table.

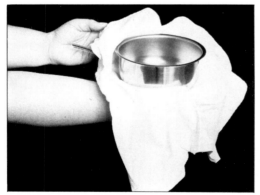

6 Pour approximately 50 ml of hydrogen peroxide solution into a basin. Then, pour sterile water into the other basin.

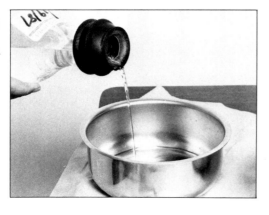

7 Put on the sterile gloves. Then, hold the two 4″x4″ gauze pads together and slit them halfway through the center with sterile scissors. Continue the procedure, using strict aseptic technique.
  Carefully inspect your patient's incision for any discharge or redness. If you see any, notify the doctor.
  Now, saturate a 4″x4″ gauze pad in hydrogen peroxide solution.

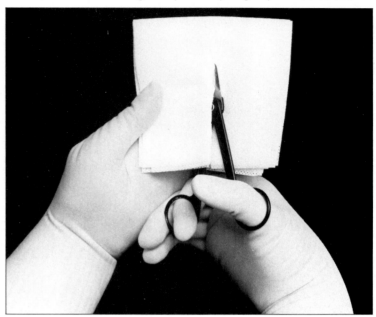

8 Starting at the top of the incision, gently wipe from top to bottom in one motion.
  Then, discard the gauze pad in the plastic bag, taking care not to touch the bag with your gloves. Repeat this procedure until you've cleaned the entire incision, using a clean gauze pad with each wiping motion.
  Note: If your patient has a T tube, carefully clean around it.

Surgical wounds

Caring for a patient with a surgical wound and drain continued

9 Next, rinse the incision site with sterile water, using the technique already described.
Using 4"x4" gauze pads, pat the area dry. Discard all used gauze pads in the plastic bag.
Now, using your nondominant hand, remove the cap from the Betadine ointment (or ask a co-worker to do this for you). Remember, this hand is no longer sterile.
Using the same hand, squeeze a small amount of ointment onto a 4"x4" gauze pad and discard the pad. Doing so ensures ointment sterility.

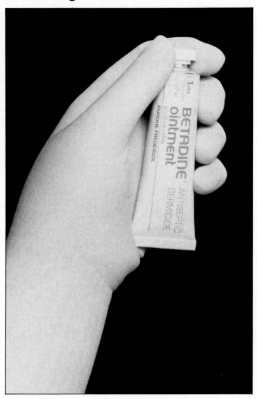

11 Cover the incision site with 4"x4" gauze pads.
Now, holding the Penrose drain with the forceps, clean around the drain, using the same technique already described.
Nursing tip: If necessary, clean around the drain with a sterile cotton-tipped applicator.
Using 4"x4" gauze pads, pat the area dry.

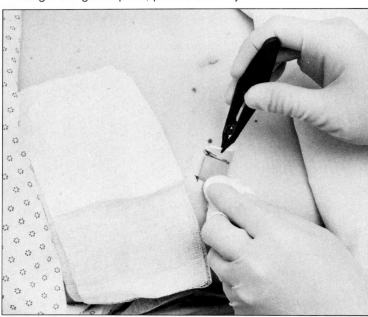

12 With your sterile scissors, cut an opening the size of the Penrose drain in the center of the Stomahesive. Then, remove the Stomahesive backing.

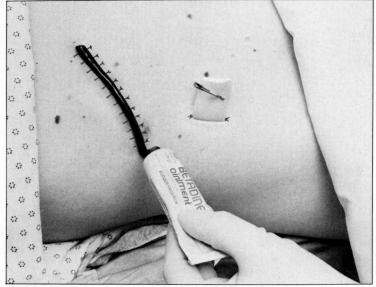

10 Squeeze ointment over your patient's entire incision, as shown in this photo. To avoid contaminating the ointment, be careful not to touch her incision with the tip of the ointment tube. Use this tube for one patient only.
Recap the ointment and put it aside. Remove your gloves and wash your hands. Put on a new pair of sterile gloves.
Note: Some doctors may order an antibiotic ointment other than Betadine.

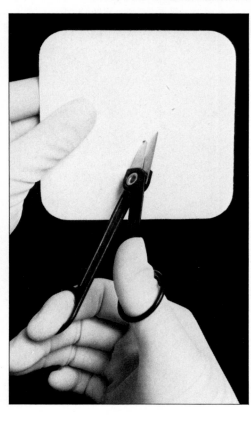

13 To alleviate skin irritation from drainage, fit the Stomahesive over the Penrose drain. Press firmly, making sure the Stomahesive sticks to your patient's skin.

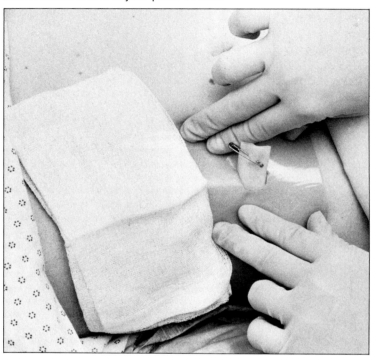

15 Put the Surgipads directly on top of the gauze pads.

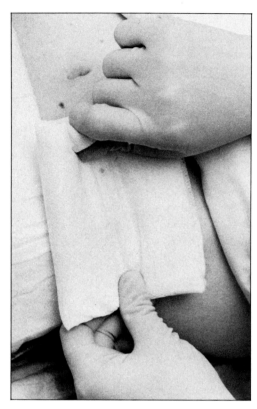

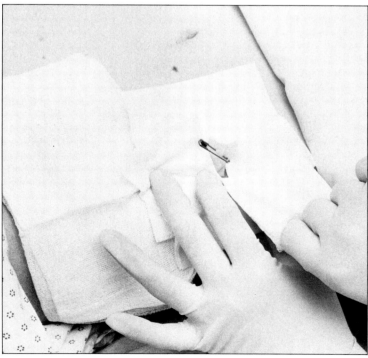

14 Grasp the two precut 4"x4" gauze pads. Fit the pads snugly around your patient's drain so the slits overlap, as shown here.

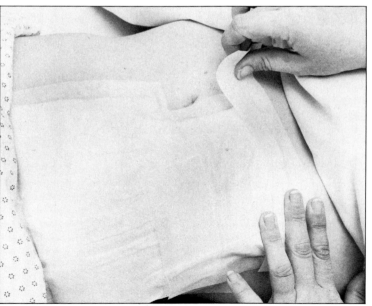

16 Tape both dressings in place. Remove your gloves and discard them in the plastic bag. Close the plastic bag with a fastener and discard it, following hospital policy. Wash and dry your hands.

Finally, document everything in your notes. Include the appearance of the incision and skin surrounding the drain, and the amount and color of drainage.

Surgical wounds

How to care for a patient with a VacuDrain™

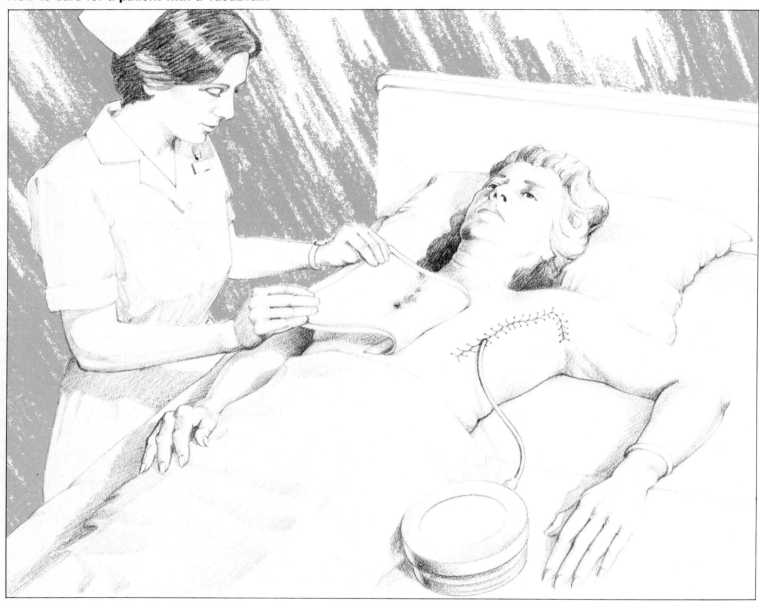

1 *Let's say 53-year-old Margaret Laslow has just returned to your floor after a mastectomy. The doctor has inserted a VacuDrain™ single-port surgical evacuator to drain her wound. You'll need to empty the evacuator container at the end of each shift, or as ordered. Do you know how? If you're unsure, follow these steps:*

First, explain the procedure to Ms. Laslow. Then, wash your hands and expose her dressing.

Examine her dressing for excessive bleeding or drainage. If you see any, suspect a dislodged or blocked drain. Notify the doctor immediately, and prepare to change Ms. Laslow's dressing, as ordered.

As you can see in these illustrations, the VacuDrain tubing is inserted directly into the wound. Make sure the perforated portion remains under your patient's skin to maintain suction.

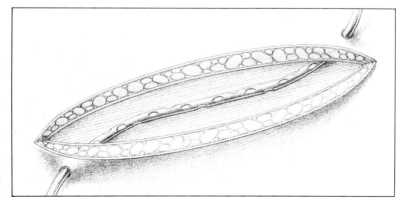

2 Now, unlock the connector attaching the drainage tubing to the evacuator container. To do this, rotate the connector a quarter-turn to the left, as shown here.

Then, remove the connector and tubing.

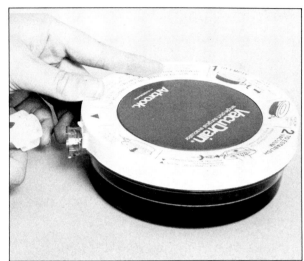

3 To protect the end of the tubing from contamination, cover it with sterile 4"x4" gauze pad and secure with a rubber band.

Through the evacuator port, empty the drainage into a measuring container, as the nurse is doing here.

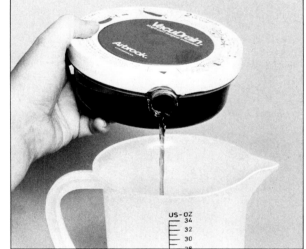

4 Now, to reestablish the vacuum, depress the center of the evacuator container top (see photo).

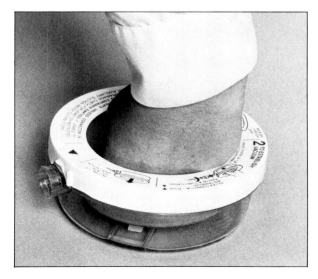

5 Keeping the top pressed down, align the red triangles on the connector and evacuator container. Push the connector over the port and rotate the connector a quarter-turn to the right. This locks the connector in place.

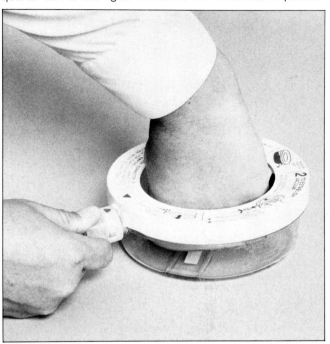

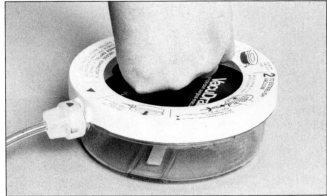

6 Next, release the top of the evacuator container to reactivate the vacuum. Place the container at a level lower than your patient's wound to ensure normal gravitational flow. To keep the container in place, you may want to loosely pin it to your patient's bedsheet. Be sure to allow enough tubing slack to permit patient free movement without dislodging tube.

Discard the drainage into the proper receptacle in the dirty utility room. Disinfect the measuring container and return it to the patient's bedside or send the container to central supply service for sterilization following hospital policy. Wash your hands.

Remember to document the drainage amount, color, odor, and consistency in your nurses' notes and in your patient's output record.

Surgical wounds

How burns affect the body

How does a burn affect the body? That depends on the depth or degree of the burn. First-degree burns, for example, partially or totally destroy the top skin layer (epidermis). As a result, the middle skin layer (dermis) and the third skin layer (subcutaneous tissue) remain unaffected. These skin layers continue to protect the patient's arteries, veins, and nerve fibers from infection. However, because of epidermal destruction, the body loses vital fluids and the patient becomes more susceptible to infection.

Second- and third-degree burns, on the other hand, destroy the epidermis, the dermis, and possibly subcutaneous tissue. These burns expose or destroy your patient's veins, arteries, and nerve fibers, increasing his infection risk.

Of course, burn therapy compromises your patient's resistance to infection, also. Why? Because caring for a patient with burns means performing several invasive therapies simultaneously. To help stabilize his condition and replace body fluids, your patient may be receiving oxygen and have an I.V., a nasogastric tube, and an indwelling (Foley) catheter. Keep in mind your patient will have open wounds (burns) requiring routine dressing changes and surgical debridement. In other words, the risk of infection increases with each type of invasive therapy your patient receives. What can you do to prevent infection? See page 147 for some special nursing guidelines.

Burn debridement: Preparing your patient

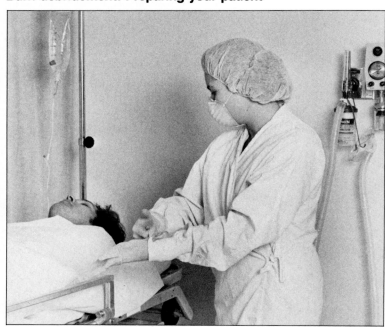

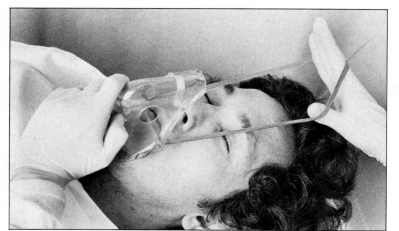

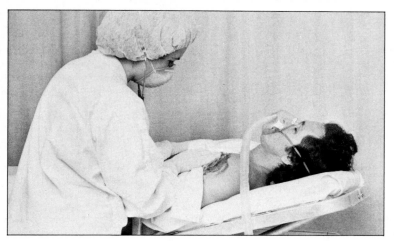

1 *Consider this: Martin Block arrives in the emergency department with severe burns on his chest and shoulders. He's received emergency care at the scene of the accident and has an I.V. in place. The doctor wants you to prepare Mr. Block for surgical burn debridement. Here's what to do:*

First, wash your hands and put on a sterile gown, cap, mask, and gloves. Explain to Mr. Block that your special garb protects his burns from contamination. Then, reassure him. Explain the procedure as you work.

Also, try to obtain as much information as possible about Mr. Block's past medical history, allergies, present physical condition, and the accident. Document the information in your nurses' notes.

2 Then, check again to be sure your patient's airway is open. Administer humidified oxygen, if necessary.

Suppose your patient has trouble breathing or shows other signs of respiratory tract damage such as singed nasal hairs or black sputum. In this case, he'll need to be intubated, following strict aseptic technique.

3 Next, take Mr. Block's blood pressure, pulse, respiration rate. Also, get an electrocardiogram. If his blood pressure is normal, elevate his head and upper torso, as shown here.

Then, assess the extent of your patient's burns. Document this information in your nurses' notes.

4 Now, remove your gloves, and discard them in a covered trash receptacle. Wash your hands and put on a new pair of sterile gloves. Then, draw a blood sample to determine type and cross-match, complete blood cell count (CBC), hemoglobin and hematocrit levels, and electrolyte balance. Also, obtain an arterial blood sample for blood gas measurements, if ordered.

Remove your gloves and discard them in a covered trash receptacle. Label the specimens and send them to the lab for immediate analysis.

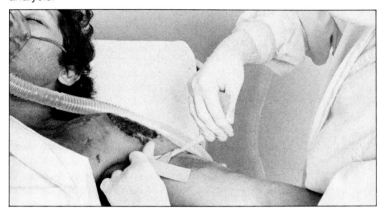

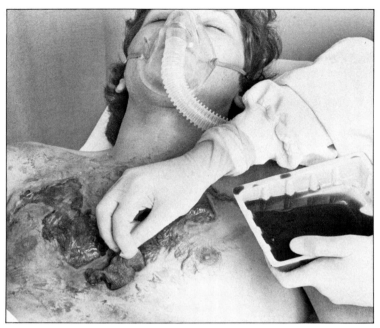

5 Wash your hands and put on a new pair of sterile gloves. Now, insert an indwelling (Foley) catheter, as ordered, following aseptic technique. Obtain a sterile urine specimen. Because your gloves are contaminated from the catheter insertion, remove and discard them.

Label and send the urine specimen to the lab for analysis.

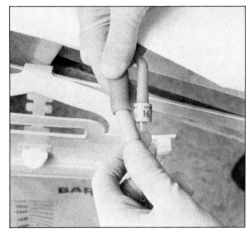

6 After you wash your hands and put on a new pair of sterile gloves, you're ready to remove gross debris from Mr. Block's burns. To do this, dip a sterile gauze pad in mild antiseptic or sterile saline solution. Then, gently cleanse the burn site, working from the center outward in one continuous motion. Discard the gauze pad and repeat this procedure on each burn.

Following doctor's orders, administer tetanus toxoid prophylactically to a patient who had a tetanus immunization within the past 10 years. For the patient who was inadequately immunized, you'll also give human tetanus immune globulin. If your patient's allergic to tetanus toxoid, notify the doctor.

Cover your patient with a sterile sheet or blanket to prevent wound contamination and additional pain from circulating air.

When Mr. Block's condition stabilizes, prepare him for a chest X-ray, according to hospital policy.

Then, notify the doctor that following Mr. Block's chest X-ray, he'll be ready for debridement.

Finally, document everything in your nurses' notes.

Caring for a patient with burns

Whenever a patient has a second- or third-degree burn, the doctor or nurse working in the burn unit may perform surgical debridement. During the procedure, he'll remove necrotic and possibly infected tissue from the burn surface, creating an open wound. Part of your patient-care responsibilities will include the wound-care guidelines, described on page 138.

But, a patient with a burn requires additional protective measures, because of his lowered resistance to infection. Follow these guidelines to provide the care he needs:
• Place your patient in a private room, an isolated area, or a burn unit, as ordered.
• Provide adequate nutrition and rest to help increase his resistance to infection.
• Wear a sterile mask, gown, gloves, and cap when providing any patient care, especially during dressing changes. If any protective

clothing becomes wet, change it immediately to protect your patient from possible contamination.
• Make sure all articles that come in contact with your patient are sterilized or highly disinfected.
• Avoid sharing equipment between patients; for example, inhalation-therapy equipment. If possible, provide individual equipment for each patient. If you must use commmon facilities, for example, during hydrotherapy, clean and disinfect the equipment immediately before and after each use, following hospital policy.
• Make sure all articles removed from your patient's bedside are cleaned and disinfected or discarded in the proper receptacle.
• To prevent the growth of microorganisms, keep the bedside pitcher covered, and change the water frequently, for example, every shift. Also, discard all opened containers of water or saline solution immediately after use.

External body openings

What's the proper way to prevent infection when caring for a patient with a urinary catheter, a tracheostomy, or a draining decubitus ulcer? Do you know how to empty a drainage bag into a graduated receptacle without causing cross-contamination? What signs indicate indwelling catheter obstruction?

If you're not sure, study this section. On these pages we'll:
• show you how to irrigate a decubitus ulcer.
• demonstrate how to safely clean around a tracheostomy cannula.
• tell you how to prevent urine reflux and decrease potential urinary tract infections.

Remember, any opening in your patient's body provides an entry port for infectious microorganisms. So reduce your patient's infection risk by reading these pages carefully.

Providing tracheostomy care

1 *Let's assume you're caring for 74-year-old Mary McNeil, a patient in your unit with a tracheostomy. As you know, you'll need to provide tracheostomy care using aseptic technique, especially if an infection exists at the tracheostomy site or the tracheostomy is new. This photostory will show you how.*

Note: For more details on tracheostomy care, see the NURSING PHOTOBOOK, PROVIDING RESPIRATORY CARE.

First, gather the equipment you'll need: a tracheostomy-care kit which includes gloves, two basins, tracheostomy bib, test tube brush, swabs, pipe cleaners, forceps, and tracheostomy ties; 4"x4" sterile gauze pads; adhesive strip; suction catheter; hydrogen peroxide solution; and sterile water or normal saline solution.

Note: Keep an extra sterile tracheostomy set at your patient's bedside for emergency reinsertion.

Explain the procedure to Mrs. McNeil.

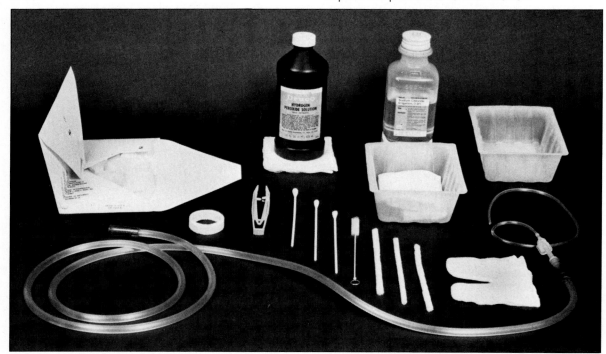

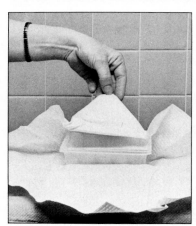

2 Wash your hands thoroughly. Then, open the kit, creating a sterile field, as the nurse is doing here.

Important: To avoid contaminating the contents, never reach across the opened kit.

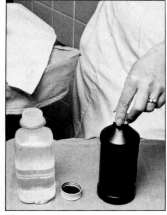

3 Now, uncap the containers of water and hydrogen peroxide solution. Place the caps—flat side down—on the table. Be careful not to touch the inside of the caps.

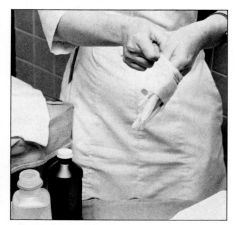

4 Next, remove the paper-wrapped gloves from the kit, and open the wrapper. Touching only the cuff, remove one glove. Hold the wrapper down to keep its outer surface from contaminating the glove.

Put on the glove.

5 Using your gloved hand, place the two basins side by side on your sterile field. Then, use your ungloved hand to pour hydrogen peroxide solution into one basin. Be careful not to touch the basin with the container. Pour the water or saline solution into the other basin.

Instruct Mrs. McNeil to take a few deep breaths, unless she's on a ventilator. Suction her airway to clear secretions. Then, ask her to take a few more deep breaths before you continue.

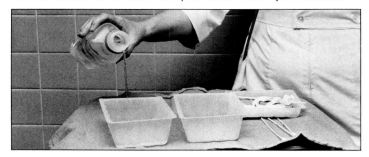

6 To clean your patient's tracheostomy tube you'll need to loosen the inner cannula with your ungloved hand. If the inner cannula locks in place, unlock it by turning it counterclockwise. But, don't remove the inner cannula at this time.

To prevent skin irritation, leave the tracheostomy bib in place, unless it's soiled. If it's soiled, use your ungloved hand to remove and discard it in a covered trash receptacle.

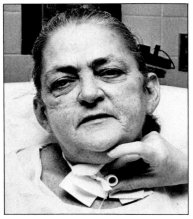

7 Now, pick up the remaining sterile glove with your gloved hand and remove the paper wrapper. Then, put on the glove.

Next, remove the loosened inner cannula by pulling it down and out. *Note:* This hand is now contaminated.

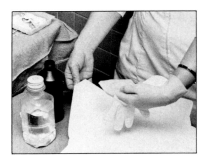

8 Immerse the inner cannula in the hydrogen peroxide solution. Use the test tube brush to clean inside the cannula, as shown here.

If the brush doesn't slide in easily, don't force it. Clean the inner cannula with a pipe cleaner instead of the brush.

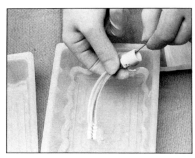

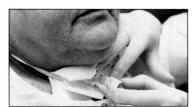

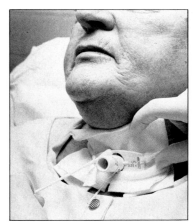

9 Now, remove the cannula from the hydrogen peroxide solution and immerse it in the sterile water or saline solution. Gently agitate the cannula for about 10 seconds and then remove it. Don't dry the cannula—simply allow the excess water or saline solution to drain into the basin. The remaining moisture will help lubricate the cannula during reinsertion.

10 With the curved portion down, reinsert the inner cannula, holding the outer cannula steady to avoid shaking it. Excessive movement may irritate your patient's trachea and cause a coughing spasm.

Lock the cannula in place.

11 Now, use a cotton-tipped swab moistened with hydrogen peroxide solution to clean around your patient's outer cannula and tracheostomy plate. To avoid contaminating the tracheostomy site, always clean from the cannula outward.

Important: Never saturate the swab. Excess solution may enter your patient's airway and trigger a coughing spasm.

When you've finished cleaning around the outer cannula and tracheostomy plate, remove your gloves and discard them in the covered trash receptacle.

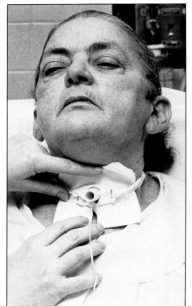

12 Next, remove and replace your patient's tracheostomy ties. Secure the ties to the plate. Replace the tracheostomy bib with a clean one, as shown here.

Then, attach an adhesive strip just below the plate to secure the trach bib. *Note:* If your patient's tracheostomy drainage is excessive, insert a precut sterile 4"x4" gauze pad from below the tracheostomy to increase drainage absorption.

Wash your hands. Remember to document the procedure and your observations in your nurses' notes.

External body openings

Providing urinary catheter care

By providing effective urinary catheter care, you'll help prevent infection and keep the catheter draining freely. Follow these guidelines:
• Always wash your hands before and after touching the catheter, tubing, or drainage bag.
• Check the catheter for proper drainage and empty the drainage bag every 8 hours using aseptic technique, or follow your hospital's policy.
• Secure the drainage bag at the side of the bed so it remains below your patient's bladder level. *Always* keep the bag off the floor to prevent contamination.
• To prevent urine flow blockage, periodically check the drainage tubing to make sure it's not kinked or looped. As you know, a blockage may cause urine reflux, leading to bladder infection or distension.
• Avoid clamping the tube. If you must clamp the tube—for example, to obtain a urine specimen—do so briefly.
• Clean your patient's perineal area at least once every day. Examine the perineal skin for signs of irritation, infection, or erosion.
• Change the catheter only when ordered, or when it's obstructed. Remember, frequent catheter changes increase the risk of infection.
• Provide adequate fluid intake to prevent residual urine pooling and possible infection.
• Give your patient ascorbic acid, as ordered, to acidify urine which inhibits microorganism growth.
• Irrigate your patient's catheter *only* as ordered. Irrigation irritates delicate tissues and may cause infection. Discard a disposable irrigation set after one use.

Using a closed drainage system

How does a closed drainage system reduce infection? By providing an unbroken junction between an indwelling (Foley) catheter and drainage tubing, as well as a sealed junction between the drainage tubing and drainage bag.

Before the closed drainage system became popular, a nurse would obtain a urine specimen or irrigate an indwelling catheter by routinely disconnecting the catheter and drainage tubing. And, each time she performed the procedure, she unfortunately created an entry port for infectious microorganisms.

However, in a closed drainage system, the catheter, drainage tubing, and drainage bag form a continuous unit. You invade this system only when absolutely necessary; for example, when an irrigation's ordered.

Another way to reduce infection is to use a catheter insertion kit with a preconnected bag. The kit helps prevent microorganisms from entering the body during catheter insertion.

How to irrigate an indwelling (Foley) catheter

1 *Your patient, 29-year-old Donald Alcorn, is recovering from kidney stone surgery. He has a Foley catheter in place. The doctor orders catheter irrigation. Do you know how to proceed? Follow these steps:*
Begin by gathering the necessary equipment: a sterile irrigation set which includes a graduated solution container, bulb or piston syringe with a rubber or plastic tip, drape, drainage-tube adapter bag, and graduated drainage basin; sterile gauze pads; povidone-iodine (Betadine) solution; irrigating solution (we're using sterile normal saline solution, at room temperature, as ordered); bed-saver pad; Hoffman clamp; and gloves.
Remember, you'll maintain strict aseptic technique during the entire procedure.

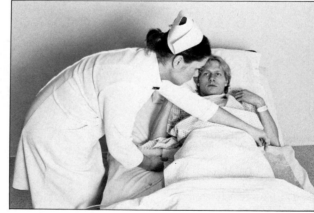

2 Wash your hands thoroughly. Then, explain the purpose of the irrigation and irrigating procedure to Mr. Alcorn. Place a drape over his pubic area to protect his privacy. Then, tuck a bed-saver pad under his buttocks and upper thighs, as shown here.
Help Mr. Alcorn into a supine position.

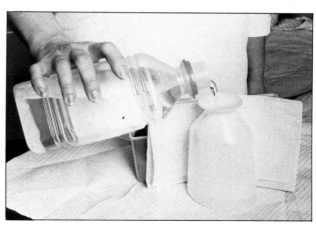

3 Using aseptic technique, unwrap your sterile equipment.
Then, open the bottle of sterile normal saline solution. Pour only as much solution as you'll need to irrigate the catheter (approximately 150 ml) into the graduated solution container. Be careful not to contaminate the inside of the solution container by touching it with the bottle.

4 Using sterile gauze pads soaked in povidone-iodine solution, thoroughly clean the catheter where it's connected to the drainage tubing.

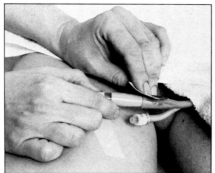

5 With a Hoffman clamp, tightly clamp the catheter above the Y-junction, as shown here.

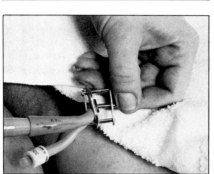

6 Now, carefully disconnect the drainage tubing from the catheter. As you hold the catheter upright to keep the end sterile, cap the tubing with a sterile plastic tip or a drainage-tubing adapter bag.

To prevent the drainage tubing from touching the floor, leave the tubing taped to your patient's leg.

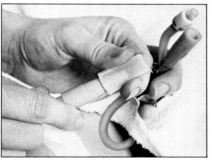

7 Position Mr. Alcorn with his knees bent and his legs abducted. Then, touching only the outside of the sterile drainage basin, place it under the catheter. Make sure the basin's secure on the bed.

Put on the sterile gloves. Then, draw about 30 ml normal saline solution into the bulb syringe. Holding the catheter steady in one hand, insert the syringe tip into the catheter. Instill 30 ml irrigation solution into your patient's bladder.

Important: To avoid bladder irritation and possible spasms, never instill the solution forcibly.

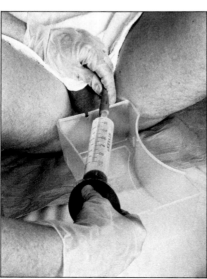

8 Now, remove the syringe and position the end of the catheter over the drainage basin. This position provides a normal gravitational flow into the basin. Make sure the end of the catheter doesn't touch the irrigation return.

Note the appearance of the returning irrigation fluid. If it's cloudy, bloody, or contains sediment, repeat the irrigation procedure until the fluid's clear, or as ordered.

Suppose no irrigation return is present. Then, stop the procedure. An obstruction or air pocket may be present. To clear the catheter, gently rotate the catheter or turn your patient from side to side. If the fluid still won't drain, notify the doctor.

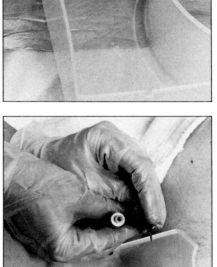

9 Wipe the distal end of the catheter and the end of the drainage tubing with povidone-iodine soaked gauze pads (see photo).

Note: In some hospitals, alcohol is used instead of povidone-iodine solution.

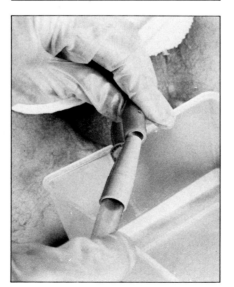

10 Next, reconnect the catheter and tubing. Discard the irrigating set and any remaining solution in the appropriate receptacles in the dirty utility room. Remove and discard your gloves in the covered trash receptacle.

Wash your hands. Then, document the procedure in your nurses' notes. Include the type and amount of irrigation solution used; the color and lucidity of the returning fluid; the presence of blood clots or sediment, if any; and your patient's tolerance to the procedure.

External body openings

How to empty a urine drainage bag

1 *Whenever you care for a patient with a closed urinary drainage system, you'll need to empty his drainage bag every 8 hours, using aseptic technique. This photostory will show you how.* Begin by washing your hands thoroughly. Then, remove the drainage tube from its protective sleeve at the bottom of the bag, as shown here. Take care not to contaminate the end of the tube by touching it with your hands or allowing it to touch the floor.

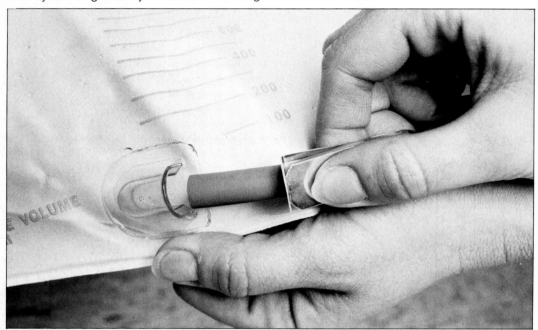

2 Now unclamp the drainage tube. Then drain the collected urine into a clean graduated receptacle, being careful not to touch the tube or your fingers to the sides of the receptacle.

Important: To prevent cross-contamination, never use the same receptacle to empty more than one drainage bag.

Make sure you hold the drainage tube above the level of the urine. In this way, you'll prevent microorganisms from being pulled up into your patient's bladder.

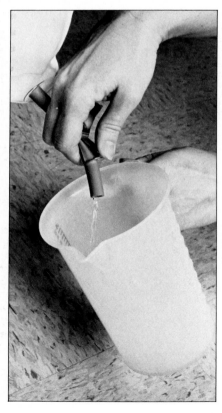

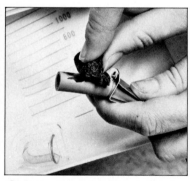

3 After the urine has drained, wipe the end of the drainage tube with povidone-iodine solution (see photo).

Clamp the tube and replace it into the drainage bag sleeve.

Empty, clean, and disinfect the graduated receptacle in the dirty utility room. Wash your hands.

Document in your notes and on your patient's intake and output record the amount of urine drained. Be sure to note the urine's color and consistency, including presence of sediment or blood.

Perineal care for the patient with an indwelling catheter

Let's say you're caring for a patient with an indwelling (Foley) catheter. As you know, one way to help prevent urinary-tract infection is to clean the perineal area and the catheter at least once a day, following hospital policy.

Begin by washing your hands thoroughly with antiseptic. Now, examine your patient's urethral meatus for signs of infection, such as erosion, inflammation, or drainage. If you see any of these signs, notify the doctor. Then, follow these steps:
• Using a washcloth, clean your patient's perineal area with a mild soap and warm water. *Note:* If your patient is male and uncircumcised, first retract his foreskin. Dry the area with a towel. Avoid using lotions, creams, or soaps containing lotions that, with prolonged use, may irritate perineal skin and create a reservoir for microorganism growth.
• Remove the tape from the catheter and drainage tubing.
• Wash your hands and put on nonsterile gloves.
• Remove any encrusted drainage on the catheter by cleaning it with soap and water. Always work outward from your patient's meatus to beyond the catheter-drainage tube junction. *Never* clean toward the meatus.

If your patient's male:
• Clean the head of your patient's penis with povidone-iodine swabs to remove secretions. To do this, wipe from the meatus outward along one side of his penis. Discard the swab and repeat the procedure until you've removed all secretions.
• Clean around the catheter-drainage tube junction with a povidone-iodine swab. To do this, hold the catheter in one hand and gently pull back on his penis approximately 1" (2.5 cm), being very careful not

to pull or tug the catheter. Discard the swab.
• Retract your patient's penis, as described above, and apply a povidone-iodine ointment to the meatus and catheter. Doing so helps destroy microorganisms that may otherwise enter your patient's body. If your patient's uncircumcised, ease his foreskin back over the glans.

If your patient's female:
• Separate her labia. Then, using a top-to-bottom motion, clean one side of the outer labia with a povidone-iodine swab. Discard the swab. Repeat this procedure on the other side of her outer labia. Now, using the same motion, clean her urethral meatus with a new swab, wiping around one side of the catheter. Discard this swab and repeat this procedure around the other side of the catheter using the remaining swabs.
• While her labia's separated, apply povidone-iodine ointment around the meatus with a cotton-tipped swab.

After the cleaning procedure, tape the catheter to your patient's leg. Take care not to pull the catheter tightly. Doing so may cause skin erosion.

Following hospital policy, tape the drainage tubing to the patient's leg. To further secure the drainage tubing, wrap adhesive tape or a rubber band around it, leaving a tab. Pin the tab to the sheet with a safety pin.

Now you're ready to remove your gloves, discard them in the proper trash receptacle, and wash your hands. Be sure to document the procedure in your notes, including any skin irritation or unpleasant odor.

Remember, perineal care may vary, so always follow your hospital's policy. For more information on caring for urologic patients, see the NURSING PHOTOBOOK IMPLEMENTING UROLOGIC PROCEDURES.

Decubitus ulcer: Changing the dressing

1 *You're caring for a patient with a decubitus ulcer. Because of the ulcer's size and depth, you decide to initiate wound and skin precautions. To treat the ulcer, the doctor has ordered silver sulfadiazine (Silvadene) ointment and dextranomer (Debrisan) applied with every dressing change. Follow these steps when changing your patient's dressing:*

First, assemble the equipment: several 4"x4" sterile gauze pads, sterile tongue depressor, Surgipad™, bed-saver pads, sterile irrigation set with normal saline solution, sterile and nonsterile gloves, and a plastic bag for discarding the soiled dressing.

Then, tell your patient what you'll be doing. Place him in a right side-lying position. Protect the bed linen with bed-saver pads. Put the plastic bag on the bed next to your patient.

Now, open the irrigation set and pour the normal saline solution into the set's container. Wash your hands and put on the nonsterile gloves. Remove the dressing from the ulcer, as shown here. Fold the soiled sides of the dressing together so they don't contaminate your gloves.

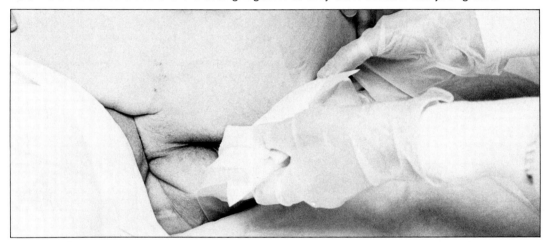

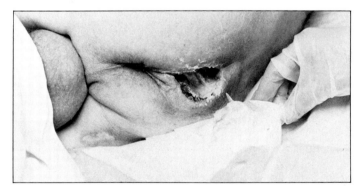

2 Carefully examine the ulcer and the dressing. Check for signs of infection, such as redness, swelling, or excessive drainage. Note the color and amount of drainage (if present). Discard the soiled dressing in the plastic bag.

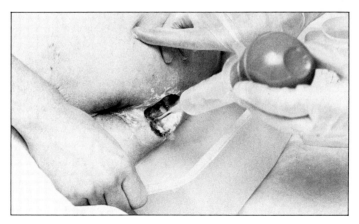

3 Now, draw up about 30 ml sterile normal saline solution into the bulb syringe. Ask a co-worker to hold the irrigating container at the ulcer's base. Then, holding the tip of the syringe about 2" (5 cm) from the ulcer, instill all the saline solution into the ulcer. This removes loose debris and previously applied medication.

Caution: To avoid contaminating the syringe and the saline solution, do not touch the syringe tip to the ulcer.

External body openings

Decubitus ulcer: Changing the dressing continued

4 Wrap a sterile gauze pad around your finger, using aseptic technique. Then, gently pat the ulcer dry, as the nurse is doing here. Discard the pad in the plastic bag. Remove your gloves and discard them in the plastic bag. Wash your hands thoroughly.

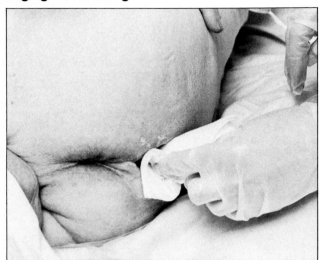

5 Next, open all your sterile supplies, creating a sterile field. Put on your sterile gloves.
   Then, holding the Silvadene container in your left hand, use the tongue depressor to scoop the Silvadene out of the container (see photo). Remember, your left hand is now contaminated.

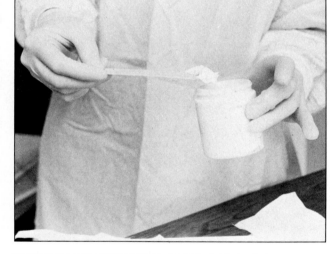

6 Using the tongue depressor, apply the ointment evenly into the ulcer, as shown here.

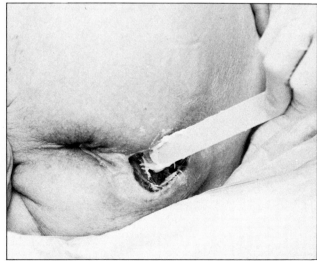

7 As you use your left hand to hold the outer surface of the sterile gauze pad at the base of the decubitus ulcer, pour the dextranomer granules into the ulcer with your right hand. Both of your hands are now contaminated.

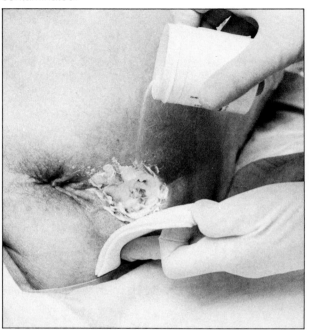

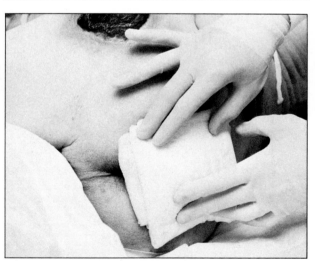

8 Cover the ulcer with fresh sterile gauze pads. Be sure to touch only the outer surface of the pads. Now, place the Surgipad over the gauze pads. Secure the dressing with nonallergenic tape.
   Now you're ready to remove your gloves. Discard them in the plastic bag. Secure the bag with a fastener and discard it in a covered trash receptacle, following hospital policy. Wash your hands.
   Document the procedure in your nurses' notes, noting drainage amount, color, and consistency, as well as the wound's appearance.

Acknowledgements

We'd like to thank the following people and companies for their help with this PHOTOBOOK:

ABBOTT LABORATORIES
North Chicago, Ill.

ACME UNITED CORPORATION
Medical Products Division
Bridgeport, Conn.
James F. Farrington
Senior Vice-President, Marketing

AMERICAN CONVERTORS
Division of American Hospital Supply Corp.
Evanston, Ill.
Joan Krase, Product Manager
Tower Products

AMERICAN CYSTOSCOPE MAKERS
Stamford, Conn.

AMERICAN HOSPITEX
Evanston, Ill.
Beth Rizer, Product Manager

AMERICAN PHARMASEAL
Glendale, Calif.
Dale Bermond, Market Manager
Diagnostic Products
Larry C. Buckelew, Market Manager
Urological Products

ANCHOR BRUSH COMPANY, INC.
Aurora, Ill.

C.R. BARD, INC.
Bard Urological Division
Murray Hill, N.J.

BARD-PARKER
Division Becton, Dickinson and Co.
Lincoln Park, N.J.

BECTON-DICKINSON
Division Becton, Dickinson and Co.
Rutherford, N.J.
Richard C. Rosencrans, Product Manager

CALGON CORPORATION
St. Louis, Mo.
William J. Evans
Hospital Products Sales Manager

CHASTON MEDICAL & SURGICAL PRODUCTS
Sales Administration
Dayville, Conn.

THE CLINIPAD CORPORATION
Guilford, Conn.
Louann Werksma, Sales Coordinator

DAVIS & GECK DEPARTMENT
Lederle Laboratories Division
American Cyanamid Company
Wayne, N.J.

C.H. DEXTER DIVISION
The Dexter Corporation
Windsor Locks, Conn.

HEALTHCO, INC.
Reading, Pa.
Al Szymborski, CMR

RAY GROSS MEDICAL
Subsidiary of Acme United Corp.
St. Louis, Mo.
Randy Mendak, Sales Manager

JOHNSON & JOHNSON PRODUCTS INC.
Patient Care Division
New Brunswick, N.J.

MARION SCIENTIFIC
Division of Marion Laboratories, Inc.
Kansas City, Mo.

M.D. INDUSTRIES, INC.
Northbrook, Ill.

MEDLINE INDUSTRIES, INC.
Northbrook, Ill.
Herb Nack, President
Accucare Division

MERCK SHARP & DOHME
West Point, Pa.

NATIONAL LABORATORIES
Lehn & Fink Industrial Products
Division of Sterling Drug, Inc.
Montvale, N.J.

PORTION-PAC CHEMICAL CORPORATION
Chicago, Ill.
Harold I. Temkin, Marketing Director

R & L PRODUCTS, INC.
Richardson, Tex.
Ronald G. Wilke, President

J. SKLAR MFG. CO., INC.
Long Island City, N.Y.

STUART PHARMACEUTICALS
Division of ICI Americas Inc.
Wilmington, Del.

SURGIKOS, INC.
Arlington, Tex.

3M
Medical Products Division
St. Paul, Minn.

VESTAL LABORATORIES
St. Louis, Mo.
Dan Gravens
Professional Products Manager

XTTRIUM LABORATORIES, INC.
Chicago, Ill.
R.E. Roche, Vice-President

MARY ELLEN BEIDEMAN, RN
Infection Control Practitioner
GEORGIA COLASANTE
Medical Technologist
ELAINE WALZ, RN
Infection Control Practitioner
Allentown and Sacred Heart
 Hospital Center
Allentown, Pa.

LORRAINE FOUNTAIN-HASSAN, RN
Infection Control Practitioner
DR. BRIAN WU
Dept. of Microbiology and Immunology
Albert Einstein Medical Center
Northern Division
Philadelphia, Pa.

ELEANOR JOHNSON, RN
Infection Control Practitioner
Quakertown Hospital
Quakertown, Pa.

Also the staffs of:

ALBERT EINSTEIN MEDICAL CENTER
Northern Division
Philadelphia, Pa.

ALLENTOWN AND SACRED HEART
 HOSPITAL CENTER
Allentown, Pa.

COMMUNITY GENERAL HOSPITAL
Reading, Pa.

QUAKERTOWN HOSPITAL
Quakertown, Pa.

ROLLING HILL HOSPITAL
 AND DIAGNOSTIC CENTER
Elkins Park, Pa.

Selected references

Books
BEING A NURSING AIDE, 2nd edition. Chicago, Hospital Research and Educational Trust, 1978.

Bennett, John, M.D. and Brachman, Philip S. (eds): HOSPITAL INFECTIONS. Boston, Little, Brown and Co., 1979.

Brunner, Lillian S.: LIPPINCOTT MANUAL OF NURSING PRACTICE, 2nd edition. New York, J.B. Lippincott Co., 1978.

Castle, Mary: HOSPITAL INFECTION CONTROL: PRINCIPLES AND PRACTICE. New York, John Wiley and Sons, Inc., 1980.

Dubay, Elaine C. and Grubb, Reba D.: INFECTION: PREVENTION AND CONTROL, 2nd edition. St. Louis, C.V. Mosby Company, 1978.

Fuerst, Elinor V., et al: FUNDAMENTALS OF NURSING: THE HUMANITIES AND THE SCIENCES IN NURSING, 5th edition. New York, J.B. Lippincott Co., 1974.

GIVING MEDICATIONS, Nursing Photobook™ Series. Horsham, Pa., Intermed Communications, Inc., 1980.

Henry, John B. and Davidsohn, Todd-Sanford: CLINICAL DIAGNOSIS & MANAGEMENT BY LABORATORY METHODS, 2 volumes, 16th edition. Philadelphia, W.B. Saunders Co., 1979.

INFECTION CONTROL IN THE HOSPITAL, 4th edition. Chicago, American Hospital Association, 1979.

Jawetz, E., et al: REVIEW OF MEDICAL MICROBIOLOGY, 13th edition. Los Altos, Ca., Lange Medical Publications, 1978.

King, Eunice M., et al: ILLUSTRATED MANUAL OF NURSING TECHNIQUES. New York, J.B. Lippincott Co., 1976.

Kunin, Calvin M.: DETECTION, PREVENTION, AND MANAGEMENT OF URINARY TRACT INFECTIONS, 3rd edition. Philadelphia, Lea & Febiger, 1979.

Lennette, Edwin H., et al (eds): MANUAL OF CLINICAL MICROBIOLOGY. Washington, DC, American Society for Microbiology, 1974.

Lewis, Laverne W.: FUNDAMENTAL SKILLS IN PATIENT CARE. New York, J.B. Lippincott, 1976.

MANAGING I.V. THERAPY, Nursing Photobook™ Series. Horsham, Pa., Intermed Communications, Inc., 1980.

Millar, Sally, et al (eds): METHODS IN CRITICAL-CARE. Philadelphia, W.B. Saunders Co., 1980.

PERFORMING GI PROCEDURES, Nursing Photobook™ Series. Horsham, Pa., Intermed Communications, Inc., 1981.

Perkins, John J.: PRINCIPLES AND METHODS OF STERILIZATION IN HEALTH SCIENCES, 2nd edition. Springfield, Ill., Charles C. Thomas, Publishers, 1978.

PROVIDING RESPIRATORY CARE, Nursing Photobook™ Series. Horsham, Pa., Intermed Communications, Inc., 1979.

Rhodes, Marie J. and Gruendemann, Barbara J.: ALEXANDER'S CARE OF THE PATIENT IN SURGERY, 6th edition. St. Louis, C.V. Mosby Co., 1978.

Smith, Alice Lorraine: PRINCIPLES OF MICROBIOLOGY, 9th edition. St. Louis, C.V. Mosby Co., 1981.

Staniew, Roger Y., Adelberg, Edward, and Ingeham, Edward A.: THE MICROBIAL WORLD. Englewood Cliffs, NJ, Prentice-Hall, Inc., 1976.

Sutton, Audrey L.: BEDSIDE NURSING TECHNIQUES IN MEDICINE AND SURGERY, 2nd edition. Philadelphia, W.B. Saunders Co., 1969.

Vander Salm, Thomas J., et al: ATLAS OF BEDSIDE PROCEDURES. Boston, Little, Brown and Co., 1979.

Periodicals

Brown, Marie S.: *What you should know about communicable diseases and their immunizations. The three R's: Part 1,* NURSING75. 5:70-72, September 1975.

Brown, Marie S.: *What you should know about communicable diseases and their immunizations. Diphtheria, pertussis, tetanus, and polio, Part 2,* NURSING75. 5:56-60, October 1975.

Brown, Marie S.: *What you should know about communicable diseases and their immunizations. Mumps, chickenpox, and diarrhea, Part 3,* NURSING75. 5:55-56, November 1975.

Furste, Wesley and Aguirre, Augusto: *Preventing tetanus,* AMERICAN JOURNAL OF NURSING. 78:834-37, May 1978.

General Recommendations on Immunization, MORBIDITY AND MORTALITY WEEKLY REPORT. 29: 81-83, 1980.

Isolation Techniques for Use in Hospitals, 2nd edition, U.S. DEPARTMENT OF HEALTH, EDUCATION AND WELFARE, CENTER FOR DISEASE CONTROL. 1975.

Koplan, Jeffrey P., Schoenbaum, S.C., Weinstein, M.C., Fraser, D.W.: *Pertussis vaccine—an analysis of benefits, risks, and costs,* NEW ENGLAND JOURNAL OF MEDICINE. 301:906-11, October 25, 1979.

McGuckin, Maryanne: *Improving your role in blood culture procedures,* NURSING76. 6:16-17 January 1976.

McGuckin, Maryanne: *The problems with respiratory tract cultures—and what you can do about them,* NURSING76. 6:19-20, February 1976.

McGuckin, Maryanne: *Urine cultures—key to diagnosing urinary tract infections,* NURSING75. 5:10-11, December 1975.

Marchiondo, Kathleen: *Collecting culture specimens,* NURSING79. 9:34-35, April 1979.

Meshelany, Cecelia., R.N., B.A.: *Post-op Wound Dressings: Your Guide to Impeccable Technique,* RN. 42:22-33, May 1979.

Morrison, Shirley T. and Arnold, Carolyn R.:*Patients with common communicable diseases—preventive measures, treatment and rehabilitation,* NURSING CLINICS OF NORTH AMERICA. 5:143-155, March 1970.

Mumps Vaccine, MORBIDITY AND MORTALITY WEEKLY REPORT. 29:87-88, 93-94, 1980.

Poliomyelitis Prevention, MORBIDITY AND MORTALITY WEEKLY REPORT. 28:510-12, 517-20, 1979.

Selekman, Janice: *Immunization: What's it all about?* AMERICAN JOURNAL OF NURSING. 80:1440-45, August 1980.

Index

A

Aerobe, 8
Alcohol
  foaming, 78
  isopropyl, 81
Anaerobe, 8
Anteroom. See *Isolation.*
Antibiotics
  administering, 109
  nurses' guide to, 106-109
  understanding, 106
Antibody, 50
Antigen, 50
Antiseptic, 77
  when to use, 80
Antitoxin, 50
Artificial active immunity, 50
  artificial passive, 50
Aseptic technique, 112

B

Bacteria, 8
Bactericidal, 77
Bacteriostatic, 77
Bed-making, 60-62
Burns. See also *Surgical wounds.*
  debridement, patient preparation, 146-147
  effect on body, 146
  patient care, 147

C

Carrier, 8
Central line
  changing dressing, 130-132
  changing tubing, 129
  insertion, 126-128
  patient care, 125
  removal, 132-133
Chicken pox. See *Varicella.*
Chlamydia, 8
Chlorhexidine gluconate, 78
Chlorine, 81
Cleaning
  soiled article (speculum), 82, 84-85
  thermometer, 66
  wheelchairs and stretchers, 65
Closed drainage system, 150
Cultures
  aerobic wound, 44-45
  anaerobic wound, 46-47
  blood, 28
  central venous pressure (CVP) catheter
    tip, 27
  cerebrospinal fluid, 26-27
  endocervical canal, 42-43
  nasopharyngeal, 18-19
  obtaining a quality specimen, 18
  sputum, 21-25
  stool, 43-44
  throat, 20-21
  urine, 30-41
Conjunctivitis, viral, work considerations, 76

D

Dakin's solution modified, 81
Decontamination, 77
Decubitus ulcer, 153-154
Diphtheria toxoid, 52
Diseases
  reportable, 72
  viral, 15-16
Disinfection, 77
Disinfectants, 81
  chlorine
  formaldehyde
  formalin
  glutaraldehyde
  iodophor
  isopropyl alcohol
  phenol
  QUATS (quaternary ammonium compounds)
DPT vaccine, 52
  diphtheria and tetanus toxoids combined, 52
  for children, 59
Drainage bag, emptying, 152

E

Ear (external), common microorganisms of, 10
Employee health
  protecting, 74
  testing, 73
Enteric precautions, 92. See also *Isolation.*
Epstein-Barr virus, 16
Eye, common microorganisms of, 10

F

Fibrinogen, 12
Formaldehyde, 81, 83
Formalin, 81, 83
Fungi, 8

G

Genitourinary system
  common microorganisms of, 10
  nosocomial infections of, 14
German measles. See *Rubella.*
Germicidal, 77
Glutaraldehyde, 81, 83
Gonorrhea, work considerations, 76

H

Hand-washing techniques, 79-80
Hepatitis, 17
  work considerations, 76
Herpes, work considerations, 76
Hexachlorophene, 78
Home care aids. See also *Self-care aids.*
  Immunizing your child, 59
Housekeeping, preventing infection, 71

I

Immunity, 50
  artificial active
  artificial passive
  natural active
  natural passive
Immunization, 50-59
  administering, 53
  basic terms, 50
  nurses' guide to, 50-52
    diphtheria and tetanus toxoids
    diphtheria and tetanus toxoids and
      pertussis vaccine (DPT)
    measles (rubeola) virus vaccine
    mumps vaccine
    poliovirus (Sabin) vaccine
    rubella virus vaccine
  schedule for children (Home care aid), 59
Impetigo, work considerations, 76
Indwelling catheter, irrigation, 150-151
Infection
  bodily reaction, 12
  chain of, 11
  defined, 8
  employee protection, 74
  food-associated, 72
  I.V.-associated, preventing, 112
  nosocomial, 12
  patient education, 71
  Salmonella, 71
  work considerations, 76
Infection-control practitioner, duties of, 73
Influenza, 16
  work considerations, 76
Injection, 53-55
  I.M. with a Tubex syringe, 55
  subcutaneous, administering, 53-55
Intestinal tract
  common microorganisms of, 10
  nosocomial infections of, 13
Intravenous (I.V.)
  adding medication via I.V. bolus, 124-125
  changing equipment, 121-122
  filter, 120
  insertion with over-the-needle catheter
    (ONC), 117-119
  insertion with winged-tip needle, 114-116
  preventing associated infections, 112
  solution, adding medication to, 122-123
Iodine, 79
Iodophor, 81
Irrigation, indwelling catheter, 150-151
Isolation
  anteroom, 93
  cart, 93
  double bagging, 102
  educating family about, 99
  educating patient about, infection control, 99
  garb
  nonsterile, donning, 95-96
    removal, 101-102
    sterile, donning, 97, 100
  patient's view of, 98
  precautions, 90

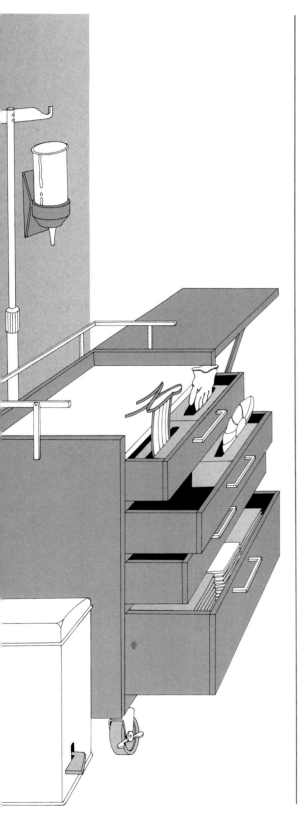

Isolation continued
  room
    setting up, 94
    terminal cleaning, 105
  transporting a patient in, 104
  types
    enteric, 92
    protective, 91
    respiratory, 91
    strict, 90
    wound and skin, 92
I.V. bolus, 124-125. See also *Intravenous.*

L

Linen. See also *Bed-making.*
  soiled, care of, 63-64
  storage procedures, 60-61
Lumbar puncture, 26

M

Measles. See *Rubeola.*
Medication. See *Intravenous.*
Microbiology, basic terms, 8
  aerobe
  anaerobe
  carrier
  colonization
  contaminant
  endotoxin
  exotoxin
  host
  pathogen
  reservoir
  source
  vector
Microorganisms
  common types, 10
  nurses' guide to, 8-9
    bacteria
    chlamydia
    fungi
    mycoplasma
    protozoa
    rickettsia
    virus
  resistant, 109
Mononucleosis, infectious, 16
  work considerations, 76
Mumps. See *Parotitis, epidemic.*
  vaccine, 52
    for children, 59
Mycoplasma, 8

N

Nasotracheal suctioning, collecting a
    sputum specimen, 23-25
Natural active immunity, 50
  natural passive, 50
Nosocomial infection, 12
  defined, 8
  identifying, 13-14
  prevention and control, 15

P

Parotitis, epidemic (mumps), 16
Pediculosis, work considerations, 76
Percutaneous procedures, understanding,
    112
Perineal care, patient with indwelling
    catheter, 152, 153
Peripheral line. See *Intravenous line.*
Pertussis vaccine, 52
Phenol, 81
Poliovirus (Sabin) vaccine, 51
  for children, 59
Protective isolation, 91. See also *Isolation.*
Protozoa, 8
Purified protein derivative (PPD). See also
    Tuberculin test.
  intradermal skin test, 74-76
    positive reaction, work considerations, 76

Q

QUATS, 81

R

Reportable diseases. See *Diseases, re-
    portable.*
Resistance
  active, 50
  passive, 50
Respiratory isolation, 91. See also *Isolation.*
Respiratory tract
  common microorganisms of, 10
  infections, work considerations, 76
  nosocomial infections of, 13
Rickettsia, 8
Rubella (German measles), 15
  vaccine, 51
    for children, 59
  work considerations, 76
Rubeola (measles), 15
  vaccine, 51
    for children, 59
  work considerations, 76

S

Sabin (Poliovirus) vaccine, 51
  for children, 59
Salmonella infection, 71
  work considerations, 76
Scabies, work considerations, 76.
Self-care aids
  collecting a urine specimen (female
      patient), 32-33
  collecting a urine specimen (male pa-
      tient), 34
Shigella, work considerations, 76
Skin, nosocomial infections of, 13
  prepping, 113
Skin-cleaning agents, identifying, 77-79
Soap
  dispenser care, 80
  types

Index

bar, 78
  dry, 78
  liquid without antiseptic, 78
  when to use, 80
Specimen. See *Cultures.*
Speculum, cleaning, 82
Sputum
  collecting a coughed specimen, 21-22
  collecting a specimen using nasotracheal
    suction, 23-25
  easing specimen collection, 21
Sterile field, creating, 136
Sterilization, 77
  double-wrapping preparation, 86-87
  liquid, 77
  methods, 83
  preparing a lightweight article for, 84-85
  wrapping guidelines, 87
Stool specimen, collecting, 43
  for ova and parasite testing, 44
Streptococcus, work considerations, 76
Stretchers, cleaning, 65
Strict isolation, 90. See also *Isolation.*
Supplies, sterile, when to replace, 87
Surgical evacuator, single-port, 144-145
Surgical wound
  nosocomial infections of, 14
  patient care, 140-143
  preventing infection, 136
  redressing
    closed wound, 136-137
    open wound, 138-139

T

Tetanus toxoid, 52
Thermometer
  bedside, 66-67
  cleaning, 66
  electronic, 68-69
  Temp-Away sheath, 68
  Tempa-Dot single-use strip, 70
Thoracentesis, 134-135
Toxin, 50
Toxoid, 50
Tracheostomy, providing care, 148-149
Tubex syringe, administering I.M. injection
  with, 55-58
Tuberculin test. See also *Purified protein
  derivative.*
  administering, 74-76
  for children, 59
Tuberculosis, work considerations, 76. See
  also *Tuberculin test.*

U

Urinary catheter care, 150
Urine specimen, collecting, 30-34
  from a nonambulatory patient, 31
  Self-care aid (female patient), 32-33
  Self-care aid (male patient), 34
  using straight catheterization
    female patient, 35-38
    male patient, 39-41

V

Vagina, common microorganisms of, 10
Varicella (chicken pox), 16
  work considerations, 76
Vascular system
  nosocomial infections of, 13
Vector, 8, 11
Viral diseases, nurses' guide to, 15-16
  epidemic parotitis
  influenza A
  infectious mononucleosis
  rubella
  rubeola
  varicella
Virus, 8

W

Wheelchairs, cleaning, 65
Wound
  closed, redressing, 137
  draining, work considerations, 76
  open, redressing, 138-139
Wound and skin precautions, 92. See also
  Isolation.

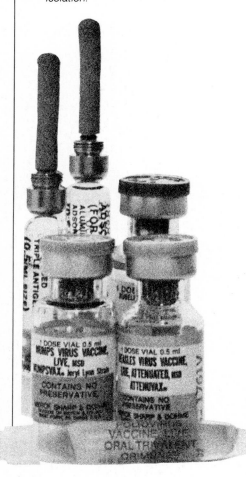